AF194404

EXPLORING THE ROLE OF ANTIVIRAL DRUGS IN THE ERADICATION OF POLIO

WORKSHOP REPORT

Committee on Development of a Polio Antiviral and
Its Potential Role in Global Poliomyelitis Eradication

Board on Life Sciences
Division on Earth and Life Studies

NATIONAL RESEARCH COUNCIL
OF THE NATIONAL ACADEMIES

THE NATIONAL ACADEMIES PRESS
Washington, D.C.
www.nap.edu

THE NATIONAL ACADEMIES PRESS   500 Fifth Street, N.W.   Washington, DC 20001

NOTICE: The project that is the subject of this report was approved by the Governing Board of the National Research Council, whose members are drawn from the councils of the National Academy of Sciences, the National Academy of Engineering, and the Institute of Medicine. The members of the committee responsible for the report were chosen for their special competences and with regard for appropriate balance.

This study was supported by Contract No. CDC-200-2000-00629 between the National Academy of Sciences and the Centers for Disease Control and Prevention (CDC) and Contract No. HQ/05/076671 between the National Academy of Sciences and the World Health Organization (WHO). The content of this publication does not necessarily reflect the views or policies of the CDC or the WHO, nor does mention of trade names, commercial products or organizations imply endorsement by the U.S. Government.

International Standard Book Number 0-309-10161-1

Cover: Upper left: Three-dimensional image of a poliovirus virion produced using an electron microscope and X-ray crystallography (courtesy of Robert Grant, Stéphane Crainic, and James Hogle, Harvard Medical School). Center: Egyptian stele with the first-known depiction of a polio victim (courtesy of Ny Carlsbert Glyptotek, Copehnagen), superimposed on the genetic sequence of the poliovirus (courtesy of Eckard Wimmer, State University of New York, Stonybrook).

Additional copies of this report are available from the National Academies Press, 500 Fifth Street, N.W., Lockbox 285, Washington, DC 20055; (800) 624-6242 or (202) 334-3313 (in the Washington metropolitan area); Internet, http://www.nap.edu.

THE NATIONAL ACADEMIES
Advisers to the Nation on Science, Engineering, and Medicine

The **National Academy of Sciences** is a private, nonprofit, self-perpetuating society of distinguished scholars engaged in scientific and engineering research, dedicated to the furtherance of science and technology and to their use for the general welfare. Upon the authority of the charter granted to it by the Congress in 1863, the Academy has a mandate that requires it to advise the federal government on scientific and technical matters. Dr. Ralph J. Cicerone is president of the National Academy of Sciences.

The **National Academy of Engineering** was established in 1964, under the charter of the National Academy of Sciences, as a parallel organization of outstanding engineers. It is autonomous in its administration and in the selection of its members, sharing with the National Academy of Sciences the responsibility for advising the federal government. The National Academy of Engineering also sponsors engineering programs aimed at meeting national needs, encourages education and research, and recognizes the superior achievements of engineers. Dr. Wm. A. Wulf is president of the National Academy of Engineering.

The **Institute of Medicine** was established in 1970 by the National Academy of Sciences to secure the services of eminent members of appropriate professions in the examination of policy matters pertaining to the health of the public. The Institute acts under the responsibility given to the National Academy of Sciences by its congressional charter to be an adviser to the federal government and, upon its own initiative, to identify issues of medical care, research, and education. Dr. Harvey V. Fineberg is president of the Institute of Medicine.

The **National Research Council** was organized by the National Academy of Sciences in 1916 to associate the broad community of science and technology with the Academy's purposes of furthering knowledge and advising the federal government. Functioning in accordance with general policies determined by the Academy, the Council has become the principal operating agency of both the National Academy of Sciences and the National Academy of Engineering in providing services to the government, the public, and the scientific and engineering communities. The Council is administered jointly by both Academies and the Institute of Medicine. Dr. Ralph J. Cicerone and Dr. Wm. A. Wulf are chair and vice chair, respectively, of the National Research Council.

www.national-academies.org

COMMITTEE ON DEVELOPMENT OF A POLIO ANTIVIRAL AND ITS POTENTIAL ROLE IN GLOBAL POLIOMYELITIS ERADICATION

Acknowledgments

THIS REPORT IS A PRODUCT of the cooperation and contributions of many people. The committee would like to thank all the speakers and participants who attended the Workshop on Development of a Polio Antiviral and Its Potential Role in Global Poliomyelitis Eradication on November 1-2, 2005, and others who provided information and input.

This report has been reviewed in draft form by persons chosen for their diverse perspectives and technical expertise in accordance with procedures approved by the National Research Council's Report Review Committee. The purpose of this independent review is to provide candid and critical comments that will assist the institution in making its published report as sound as possible and to ensure that the report meets institutional standards of objectivity, evidence, and responsiveness to the study charge. The review comments and draft manuscript remain confidential to protect the integrity of the deliberative process. We wish to thank the following for their review of this report:

Craig Cameron, Pennsylvania State University
Walter Dowdle, The Task Force for Child Survival and Development
Christopher D. Earl, BIO Ventures for Global Health
Diane E. Griffin, Johns Hopkins Bloomberg School of Public Health
James M. Hogle, Harvard Medical School
Karla Kirkegaard, Stanford University School of Medicine
Amy K. Patick, Pfizer

Bert L. Semler, University of California, Irvine School of Medicine
P. Frederick Sparling, University of North Carolina School of Medicine

Although the reviewers listed above have provided constructive comments and suggestions, they were not asked to endorse the conclusions or recommendations, nor did they see the final draft of the report before its release. The review of this report was overseen by Donald S. Burke of the Johns Hopkins Bloomberg School of Public Health and Nicole Lurie of the RAND Corporation. Appointed by the National Research Council, they were responsible for making certain that an independent examination of this report was carried out in accordance with institutional procedures and that all review comments were carefully considered. Responsibility for the final content of this report rests entirely with the author committee and the institution.

Contents

SUMMARY   1

**1   AN OVERVIEW OF THE POLIO ERADICATION
     CHALLENGE**   7

2   PUBLIC HEALTH CONSIDERATIONS   13

**3   POTENTIAL BIOLOGICAL TARGETS OF
     POLIO ANTIVIRAL DRUGS**   19
     Synopsis of Poliovirus Pathogenesis and Replication, 20
     Targets for Polio Antivirals, 23
     Basic Research Needs, 33

**4   DEVELOPMENT OF ANTIVIRAL DRUGS FOR
     POLIOVIRUS**   35
     Potential Hurdles to Address at the Outset, 36
     Identifying and Optimizing Potential Polio Antiviral Drugs, 37
     Clinical Development, 41
     The Importance of Developing More Than One Antiviral Drug, 43
     Timelines and Costs, 44

5   IMPLEMENTATION AND RECOMMENDATIONS   47
     Recommedations, 48

REFERENCES   **51**

APPENDIXES

A	Statement of Task	**61**
B	Committee Biographical Sketches	**63**
C	Workshop Agenda and Participant List	**69**

Summary

WHEN THE GLOBAL POLIO ERADICATION CAMPAIGN was launched in 1988, poliovirus caused more than 350,000 cases of paralytic disease annually in more than 125 countries. By 2003, only 784 cases of poliomyelitis were reported in a total of six countries (Aylward et al. 2005). This tremendous public health achievement—accomplished through the cooperation of international organizations, individual governments, private organizations and hundreds of thousands of volunteers—has vastly reduced the public health burden once imposed by paralytic polio. The final steps in the eradication of polio, however, pose a challenge.

The tool that has been crucial to the eradication effort can itself become a persistent source of poliovirus in the community. The oral polio vaccine, originally developed by Albert Sabin, contains weakened versions of each of the three strains of poliovirus. It is relatively inexpensive to produce and can be given by mouth. The vaccine viruses grow in the recipient's intestines, causing a symptomless infection in the immunocompetent host that stimulates highly protective, enduring immunity to disease. The vaccine viruses can also spread to people who are in contact with the recipient, increasing the coverage of an immunization campaign. This last characteristic, however, now represents a serious problem. As the vaccine strains spread from person to person, they can mutate and reacquire the ability to cause paralytic disease. If the percentage of the population that is immunized is not kept very high, the vaccine-derived paralytic polioviruses can circulate among the unimmunized population and may cause new outbreaks of paralytic disease. The ability of viruses derived from the oral vaccine to persist in the population poses a substantial challenge to the final stages of eradication.

Another problem is that oral polio vaccination of individuals with immune deficiencies can result in persistent infections, if not disease, in which the vaccine recipient can shed highly neurovirulent virus over extended periods of time. Attempts to cure these individuals have so far been unsuccessful. The known number of persistently infected individuals is exceedingly small, but the actual number of such shedders globally cannot be assessed at the present time.

As long as oral polio vaccine continues to be administered routinely, the spread of vaccine-derived poliovirus is not a problem. Once wild poliovirus is eradicated, an achievement that is anticipated by the global polio eradication campaign authorities in the next few years, the current plan is to discontinue universal administration of oral polio vaccine. Aside from the difficulty of maintaining financial and political support for vaccinating against a virus that seems to have disappeared and is no longer causing disease, the oral vaccine itself causes paralytic disease in a very small number of recipients—about 1-2 per million. At some point, the continued administration of the oral vaccine may pose a greater risk than does the wild virus. As the time approaches when wild poliovirus is expected to be eradicated, a strategy is needed to deal with the ramifications of discontinuing universal vaccination with the oral polio vaccine.

At the request of the Centers for Disease Control and Prevention and the World Health Organization, a committee was established by the National Research Council to organize a workshop to evaluate whether an antiviral drug against poliovirus would be helpful in the final stages of the global polio eradication campaign. The committee was not asked to evaluate the plan to discontinue universal vaccination with oral polio vaccine or other aspects of the post-eradication plans developed by the agencies. Rather, the committee was asked only to address the following issues:

- The feasibility and appropriateness of using a polio antiviral drug in the post-eradication era
- The properties a polio antiviral compound would need in order to meet the goals of the eradication program
- The most promising targets for polio antiviral drug development
- A comparison of different approaches to polio antiviral drug development, including an assessment of the required scientific expertise, infrastructural needs, risks, obstacles, and relative costs

This report is based on discussions at the workshop, which was held in Washington, DC, on November 1-2, 2005. The workshop was attended by 30 people in addition to the seven committee members. The full statement of task, committee members' biographies, workshop agenda, and participant list are included as Appendixes A-C.

In the event that universal vaccination with oral polio vaccine is discontinued, the committee concludes that it would be extremely useful and possibly essential to develop another tool to control outbreaks of poliomyelitis in an increasingly immunologically susceptible world. The availability of an antiviral drug would provide the public health community much-needed flexibility in reacting to post-oral vaccine outbreaks. The models that have been developed to evaluate the likelihood of post-eradication outbreaks suggest that outbreaks are very likely in the first few years after cessation of universal vaccination but that the risk will then rapidly decline. Discussions at the two-day workshop were not in sufficient depth to allow the committee to evaluate the quality of these models. The committee notes, however, that there is considerable uncertainty about some of the parameters used in the models. Interrupting the final chains of transmission may prove more difficult than these models suggest. The committee concludes that it is not currently possible to predict exactly how the eradication of wild polioviruses and the residual problem of vaccine-derived polioviruses will play out. Among possible scenarios, it is possible that vaccine-derived strains will persist and continue to cause outbreaks longer than currently projected. Under such circumstances, continuing to respond to outbreaks with live polio vaccines may become undesirable. Using inactivated polio vaccines may be preferred, but may not be sufficient. The immunity provided by the inactivated vaccine prevents paralytic disease by blocking spread of the virus from the intestinal tract to the central nervous system, but does not protect against intestinal poliovirus infection and, ergo, viral replication. Therefore it is ill-suited to preventing the spread of poliovirus infections, especially in countries where water supplies are unhygienic and vaccination is carried out by periodic campaigns rather than as part of routine medical care. A drug that prevents infection and spread during the time the inactivated vaccine is being administered might be required for use in concert with the inactivated vaccine to contain outbreaks.

The committee concludes that it would be appropriate to use an antiviral drug to protect vaccine recipients from poliovirus infection and to limit spread until immunity can be assured. Such a drug would have to be extremely safe, especially for children, as well as stable and easy to use. It would have to be active against all poliovirus types and possibly against non-polio enteroviruses. The success of an antiviral drug strategy will also depend on cost, timely distribution and compliance. Therefore an antiviral program will require not only the development of the antiviral drug itself, but also detailed plans for how it will be deployed and how compliance with the recommended usage will be ensured.

There are reasons for optimism: the poliovirus has been well characterized biologically and presents a number of vulnerable targets for antiviral drugs, and promising lead molecules have already been identified for two of these targets. The committee recommends that the development of these compounds be explored further. Indeed, the committee identified several additional promising targets for potential polio antiviral drugs and there are, in fact, others that were brought to the committee's attention subsequent to the workshop. Since workshop discussions were not sufficiently comprehensive to justify recommending a particular molecule for development, the report describes some of the advantages and disadvantages of each of the targets discussed at the workshop. The committee recommends that a secondary research effort be continued into targets not chosen for immediate development in order to ensure that there are additional compounds entering the development pipeline. Continued basic research into poliovirus will be necessary to support the development effort.

The committee recommends the formation of a multidisciplinary steering group to oversee the development of polio antiviral drugs. Proving the safety and efficacy of a novel polio antiviral drug will require a well-conceived and well-conducted development and testing strategy, including studies using animal models and large clinical safety trials. The choice of the best targets, the formulation of a credible development plan and the early solicitation of advice from regulatory authorities should be undertaken by the steering group, since detailed justification of the plan will be extremely important to attract the investment needed.

The development of one or more antiviral drugs against poliovirus, although expensive, serves as an insurance policy that provides an additional means of reacting to repeated outbreaks due to continued circulation of vaccine-derived strains, should they occur. Furthermore, the existence of such antiviral drugs, in combination with stockpiled vaccine, would provide the ability to respond to a future accidental or intentional reintroduction of poliovirus. The consequences of a laboratory accident or a bioterrorist attack with poliovirus will grow increasingly severe after universal vaccination has ceased. Experience with the development of drugs against other viruses suggests that it will take at least several years to develop effective polio antiviral drugs and therefore that it would be unwise to wait until the above scenarios play out. If the need for such a drug arises, it will be too late to initiate the drug development program. The committee recognizes that marshalling the resources to develop antiviral drugs against polio will be challenging. Drug development requires a large, long-term investment with an unsure outcome. However, the public health burden of paralytic polio that has been lifted as a result of the eradication effort is enormous and the recommended investment in drug development can be seen as the capstone to past investments in polio eradication. The committee concludes that it is important to ensure that past investment in the eradication effort be protected and therefore that it would be prudent to develop at least one, but preferably two, polio antiviral drugs as a supplement to the tools currently available for the control of poliomyelitis outbreaks in the post-eradication era.

1

An Overview of the
Polio Eradication Challenge

At the request of the Centers for Disease Control and Prevention (CDC) and the World Health Organization (WHO), a committee was established by the National Research Council to organize a workshop to evaluate whether an antiviral drug against poliovirus would be helpful in the final stages of the global polio eradication campaign. The committee was not asked to evaluate the plan to discontinue universal vaccination with oral polio vaccine (OPV) or other aspects of the post-eradication plans developed by the agencies. Rather, the committee was asked only to address the following issues:

- The feasibility and appropriateness of using a polio antiviral drug in the post-eradication era
- The properties a polio antiviral compound would need in order to meet the goals of the eradication program
- The most promising targets for polio antiviral drug development
- A comparison of different approaches to polio antiviral drug development, including an assessment of the required scientific expertise, infrastructural needs, risks, obstacles, and relative costs

This report is based on discussions at the workshop, which was held in Washington, DC, on November 1-2, 2005. The workshop was attended by 30 people in addition to the seven committee members. The full statement of task, committee members' biographies, workshop agenda, and participant list are included as Appendixes A-C.

The situation facing public health authorities who are responsible for the polio eradication effort is very complex and much effort has gone into developing current plans. The two-day workshop held by this committee was not designed to evaluate those plans and the description that follows should not be construed either as endorsement or criticism. Instead, this section is provided to acquaint the reader with the assumptions that the committee used in coming to its recommendations regarding the development of antiviral drugs against polio.

The successful campaign to eradicate smallpox stands as one of history's greatest public health achievements. It has served as an inspiration for the huge commitment needed to eradicate other infectious diseases. Lessons learned from the smallpox campaign have informed the choice of diseases to target and the strategy behind later eradication campaigns. In 1988, the WHO identified poliomyelitis as a disease that merited global eradication and met the basic biological conditions for potentially successful eradication (Fenner et al. 1988):

- The microbial agent infects only humans.
- Humans are the only reservoir for the microbial agent.
- The infection induces life-long immunity.
- There is a tool or intervention that effectively interrupts the chain of transmission of the infectious agent from one individual to another.

OPV has been highly successful in interrupting the transmission of wild poliovirus through most of the eradication campaign; but as the final stages approach, the final condition is proving problematic. OPV, which contains live, attenuated versions of all three poliovirus types, does induce enduring immunity, but can itself transmit polioviruses to nonimmune people and, rarely, (1-2 per million recipients) causes paralytic disease. As long as OPV is used, new chains of transmission can be initiated among susceptible people. Interruption of these final challenging chains of transmission may require a different approach.

When the global polio eradication campaign was launched in 1988, poliovirus caused more than 350,000 cases of paralytic disease annually in more than 125 countries. By 2003, only 784 cases of poliomyelitis were reported in a total of 6 countries (Aylward et al. 2005). The tremendous success of this program occurred in spite of the fact that polio has proven in several ways more difficult to eradicate than smallpox. In contrast with the characteristic rash of smallpox, the vast majority of poliovirus infections are subclinical; surveillance is therefore more difficult, as is defining the extent of spread. Smallpox spreads by face-to-face contact, but poliovirus is transmitted by fecal-oral transmission and can survive in local water supplies for weeks. Furthermore, OPV must be kept refrigerated and administered repeatedly in contrast with the single inoculation needed with the highly stable smallpox vaccine. In spite of these challenges, the strategy of populationwide National Immunization Days (NIDs) held a month or two apart and repeated at various intervals has succeeded in reducing the burden of poliomyelitis to the point where eradication appears attainable. Despite the earlier setbacks in 2004-2005, transmission of wild poliovirus had been interrupted in all but a few countries (esp. Nigeria, Somalia, Ethiopia, Yemen, Indonesia, and India) by the end of 2005. The setbacks were the consequence of cessation of vaccination in northern Nigeria; type 1 virus spread to a dozen countries, some of which had been polio-free for as long as 10 years (WHO 2005).

Thus, the final steps in eradicating polio pose a challenge that was not faced in the smallpox campaign. OPV, which has been so successful in interrupting the transmission of wild poliovirus, can initiate new chains of transmission. Vaccine-derived polioviruses (VDPVs) can evolve in two ways. In areas where vaccine coverage rates are low and an OPV recipient may come into contact with many susceptible people, infection of a susceptible contact with excreted OPV may initiate a continuing chain of transmission of the virus (which is then called a circulating-vaccine derived poliovirus or cVDPV) among other susceptible people (Kew et al. 2004). Less common, but of major importance, is the prolonged excretion of VDPV by patients who have B-cell immune deficiencies (such as agammaglobulinemia, common variable immunodeficiency, and severe combined immunodeficiency), whose chronically excreted virus is labeled iVDPV (Kew et al. 1998). Although some of these immunodeficient patients develop vaccine-associated paralytic polio (VAPP), others may excrete iVDPV for years while remaining totally asymptomatic (MacLennan et al. 2004; Martin et al. 2004). As the vaccine-derived viruses replicate, either by circulation through susceptible people in the population or in immunocompromised people, they accumulate mutations and can reacquire the ability to infect the central nervous system (CNS) and cause paralytic disease. Reversion to highly neurovirulent phenotypes is particularly pronounced in OPV-derived strains that have recombined with non-polio

TABLE 1 Recent Outbreaks of Paralytic Polio Caused by cVDPVs (Sutter 2005)

Country	Year	Number of Known Cases
Indonesia	2005	31
Madagascar	2002, 2005	5, 2
China	2004	2
Cambodia*	2003	3
Philippines	2001	3
Hispaniola	2000	21
Egypt	1988-1993	32

*Arita et al. 2005.

enteroviruses, specifically C-cluster coxsackie viruses (Kew et al. 2005, 2004). Transmission and neurovirulence phenotypes of these circulating viruses (cVDPVs) are indistinguishable from wild polioviruses. In the context of a fully immunized population, the presence of VDPVs is not a threat, but if rates of immunization decline, these strains can initiate new chains of transmission of virulent poliovirus. There have been several outbreaks of paralytic polio caused by such VDPV strains in insufficiently immunized populations (Table 1).

The ability of OPV-derived viruses to persist in the population poses a substantial challenge to the final stages of eradication. However, continuing the use of OPV indefinitely, which could prevent the spread of cVDPV, is problematic. OPV administration must be maintained at nearly universal levels to prevent outbreaks of VDPV, as the examples in Table 1 demonstrate. It will be difficult to maintain financial and political support for repeated campaigns against a virus that is no longer seen to be causing disease. Also, OPV itself, as mentioned previously, causes paralytic disease in a very small number of the children to whom it is administered, so at some point after the eradication of wild poliovirus the continued administration of OPV may be seen to pose a greater risk than does the wild virus.

The final stages of polio eradication therefore pose a dilemma. On the one hand, if OPV use can be discontinued, the source of live polioviruses for vaccine-derived outbreaks is eliminated, as is the risk of VAPP. On the other hand, OPV cessation results in a cohort of children and probably some young adults who will be vulnerable to infection by any remaining wild polioviruses or by cVDPV. In wealthy countries, the response to this dilemma has been to cease administration of OPV and to administer instead an inactivated poliovirus vaccine (IPV). The immunity provided by IPV does not protect against intestinal poliovirus infection, but it does block spread of the virus from the intestinal tract to the central nervous system and thus prevents paralytic disease (Kew et al. 1998). Therefore, a cVDPV will not cause paralytic disease in a population protected by IPV. Polioviruses may, however, be able to circulate in such a population. This characteristic means that an IPV-based immunization strategy may not be effective in interrupting the spread of polioviruses in poor countries that do not provide immunization on a routine basis in infancy and do not have reliably clean water supplies. Furthermore, IPV, which must be injected, is currently more expensive and difficult to administer than OPV. An additional disadvantage of using IPV is that it is prepared from highly virulent poliovirus strains, whose continued production would grow increasingly risky as immunization levels declined. However, continued research may lead to new IPV candidates with novel effective and inexpensive delivery methods.

If it is desirable to find a way to stop having to administer OPV universally and indefinitely, and universal administration of IPV is not a suitable alternative at the present time, how are the final challenges of polio eradication to be overcome? As the time approaches when wild poliovirus is expected to be eradicated, a strategy is needed to deal with the ramifications of discontinuing universal vaccination with OPV.

The desirability of simultaneously ending the use of OPV worldwide is clear; the risk of spread of cVDPVs from areas still using the vaccine to those that have stopped is otherwise too high. Even with simultaneous cessation, it is recognized that cVDPVs will almost certainly emerge (Kew et al. 2005). The risk of initiating a new chain of transmission is expected to decline rapidly as the last round of children to receive OPV stop shedding the virus. At the same time, the proportion of the population susceptible to infection will begin to grow as soon as OPV use ends. There are approximately 350,000 births in the world every day, and over 130 million births annually. By 4 years after the cessation of OPV use, the proportion of the population lacking any immunity to poliovirus will approach 15-20% in many developing countries. Notably, the 0-4 year-old age group makes up from approximately 6% of the population in developed countries to almost 20% in some poor countries (Census Bureau 2005).

The current strategy calls for intensive surveillance so that any emergence of cVDPV is detected rapidly. The use of monovalent OPV (mOPV, containing only the poliovirus type implicated in the outbreak) has proved effective in extinguishing outbreaks in the past and therefore is the expected strategy for containing outbreaks in the post-OPV era (CDC 2005a). However, recent responses to cVDPV outbreaks have occurred in a well-immunized surrounding population, and this would continue to be true in the first years after OPV use has ceased. Models suggest that massive local intervention with mOPV would be capable of ending an outbreak without leaving enough susceptible people to sustain new chains of transmission (Duintjer Tebbens et al. 2005). Workshop discussions were not detailed enough to allow the committee to rigorously evaluate the models on which current eradication plans are based, but the committee believes that there are still too many unknowns to predict with certainty how the post-eradication scenario will unfold. The recent discovery of an iVDPV in five unvaccinated Amish children in Minnesota, 6 years after the discontinuation of OPV use in the United States and in the face of nearly universal vaccination with IPV in the surrounding population, suggests that the last chains of transmission of vaccine strains will be difficult to detect and terminate (CDC 2005b).

2

Public Health Considerations

Tʜᴇ ᴄᴏᴍᴍɪᴛᴛᴇᴇ ᴄᴏɴsɪᴅᴇʀᴇᴅ ʜᴏᴡ an antiviral drug could be applied in the field to further the goal of global polio eradication. The committee recognizes that a drug that inhibits poliovirus replication *in vivo* has the potential to be used for *prevention* of infection or for *treatment* of infected patients. Because the challenges to polio eradication in the immediate post-OPV era are different from those in the more distant future, more than 3 years after OPV cessation (Aylward and Cochi 2004), each of these timeframes is considered individually. The utility of antiviral drugs for the treatment of chronic shedders, the potential sources of iVDPV, is addressed separately.

Production of a drug that *prevents* infection or reduces viral shedding among those who are infected would be the major goal of an antiviral drug development program in support of global polio eradication. A drug designed for prevention of infection would require an oral formulation that is safe, effective, affordable, and unlikely to induce transmission of resistant polioviruses. An ideal prophylactic drug would require only one, or at most two doses per day for optimal compliance. Its use would be limited to distribution by public health authorities in the event of an outbreak of wild type poliovirus or vaccine-derived poliovirus (VDPV) infection. When given to all who are at risk of infection as the sole strategy, an antiviral agent given to those with current (but unidentified) poliovirus infection might prevent paralytic disease in recipients and reduce the risk of transmission of the outbreak strain to susceptible contacts. However, the committee concludes that it is most likely that an antiviral drug would be used as a supplement to vaccination in order to prevent infection.

In the **first 2-3 years after OPV cessation**, response to outbreaks of cVDPV is expected to consist of comprehensive, regional mOPV distribution (Aylward and Cochi 2004). Because the immune response to a live vaccine depends on replication of the vaccine virus in the gastrointestinal tract, concomitant administration of a potent antiviral drug would interfere with the induction of immunity. Therefore, when OPV is used for outbreak control, the role of an antiviral drug might be quite limited. If sufficiently safe and inexpensive, such a drug might be used by public health authorities to control spread of live polioviruses—both the virulent outbreak virus and OPV viruses—in unaffected areas that surround the outbreak zone. The drug supply would need to be very large and the logistics of distributing the drug would be complex, potentially draining resources from the areas affected by the outbreak.

The risk of an outbreak of cVDPV **more than 3 years after OPV cessation** is thought to be low (Duintjer Tebbens et al. 2005), but the consequences could be severe, in that the number of susceptible children would by then be substantial. It is during the period more than 3 years after OPV cessation that the committee concludes that an antiviral drug may be most useful. If such an outbreak occurs and it is undesirable to reintroduce live poliovirus to control it, IPV could be used as an alternative. IPV is safe and carries no risk either of VAPP or of initiating a cVDPV chain of transmission. However IPV does not induce a mucosal immune response and thus is less effective in interrupting transmission of polioviruses. By itself, IPV may not induce immunity quickly enough to stop an outbreak. Use of an antiviral drug in conjunction with IPV would protect vaccine recipients from poliovirus infection until IPV-induced immunity can be assured. Virtually all studies with the currently available IPV vaccines confirm that at least two doses are required to achieve seroconversion in more than half the vaccinees. Actual seroconversion rates vary, not only with the number of doses, but also with the interval between doses and with age (Sormunen et al. 2004; Simoes et al. 1985). Simoes et al. showed that IPV containing 40, 8, and 30 D antigen units for serotypes 1, 2, and 3, respectively, induced seroconversion rates of 96%, 80%, and 96% 4 weeks after the second dose, if two IPV doses were administered a month apart (Simoes et al. 1985). These rates are slightly lower than rates observed after a 2-month dose interval but it is likely that the shortest effective interval between IPV doses would be chosen for purposes of outbreak control.

To be effective in supplementing an outbreak response with IPV, a polio antiviral drug would have to exhibit the following characteristics:

- *Extreme safety*—especially for young children because the drug would be given to young IPV recipients and taken daily for 4-6 weeks.
- *Oral administration*—in liquid form because it must be available for infants and young children.
- *Once, or at most twice, daily dosing*—to encourage compliance.
- *Stability*—to allow production and stockpiling before outbreaks occur.
- *High activity against all poliovirus types*—specifically,
  —*In uninfected patients* to prevent infection or markedly reduce virus shedding if infected.
  —*In already infected patients* to reduce infection to a level where the likelihood of transmission to susceptible contacts is very low and, ideally, to prevent progression to the central nervous system (CNS). Halting the progression of the disease once it has reached the CNS may not be possible.

Of course, the success of an antiviral drug strategy will also depend on factors unrelated to the agent's pharmacological properties, efficacy, and safety. These include the cost of the drug, the expense of distribution, the ability to identify the target population and distribute the drug in a timely manner, and compliance among those who are given the drug. Therefore an antiviral program will require not only design, manufacture, and testing of an antiviral, but also detailed plans that include criteria for employment of the drug, a distribution strategy, and innovative ways of enhancing compliance.

It is not possible to ignore the ease with which RNA viruses such as poliovirus develop resistance. In a setting in which a drug and a virus co-exist for any amount of time—for example, when a drug is given continuously to control a chronic viral infection, such as HIV—the development of resistance is virtually certain. In the prophylactic setting described above, it is anticipated that the great majority of recipients will not be infected with poliovirus at all; in these patients, the drug will not be exerting selective pressure on the virus. In patients who are already infected (but asymptomatic) when they receive the drug, it will be important that the drug work quickly enough for the patient to be unlikely to pass on the virus (if it is passed on, it might come under selective pressure in successive patients, increasing the chances of developing resistance).

Although development of a drug with *therapeutic* efficacy would not be the main objective of an antiviral development program to aid eradication of poliomyelitis, it is possible, if not likely, that a prophylactic drug would have the potential to ameliorate disease or reduce the risk of developing disease in persons infected with poliovirus. An antiviral drug, if available, would probably be given to patients who had acute paralytic poliomyelitis in the hope of favorably altering the natural course of neurological disease, although it is unlikely that true therapeutic efficacy could ever be measured with confidence. A therapeutic drug might also have both personal and public health benefits when made available to treat immunodeficient persons known to be persistently infected with live poliovirus. The number of such chronic shedders is thought to be extremely small; fewer than 30 have ever been identified and only 3 are known to be alive now (Halsey et al. 2004). All 3 of these patients live in developed countries that have replaced or will someday replace OPV with IPV. If the number of chronic shedders turns out to be higher than now expected, especially in poor countries, they could become a source of live virus in countries that cease vaccination and a treatment that could reduce or eliminate shedding would provide a significant public health benefit.

It is recognized that the difficulty of identifying all chronic virus shedders, particularly in developing countries, may impede this application of an antiviral drug. With so few patients, it would be virtually impossible to complete a well-designed clinical trial to demonstrate clinical benefit for either acutely infected or chronically infected persons. Long-term use of the drug in chronic shedders could theoretically lead to development of resistant virus. Therefore, it would be ideal to have more than one antiviral drug available, so that combination therapy could be used to discourage the emergence of resistance in patients who might take the drugs for extended periods. Because of the very small number of such patients, the difficulty of demonstrating the efficacy of such a compound and the likelihood that drugs that would be effective for prophylactic use in normal populations might not be as effective in the immunocompromised, the committee does not recommend that effort be concentrated on developing drugs to cure chronic shedders. However, it is anticipated that any antiviral drugs developed for prophylaxis may also have some efficacy in this small patient population.

If, as currently planned, universal vaccination with OPV is discontinued, it would be extremely useful and may, in fact, be essential to have additional tools to control outbreaks of poliomyelitis in an increasingly susceptible world. The availability of an antiviral drug that either prevents infection altogether or decreases shedding of the virus to levels that prevent transmission would give the public health community much-needed flexibility in reacting to post-vaccination outbreaks.

3

Potential Biological Targets of
Polio Antiviral Drugs

T HE PREVIOUS CHAPTER DELINEATED several qualities that a successful polio antiviral drug would need to have to be valuable in the eradication program. As part of the "ideal" drug profile (low cost, safety, preference for oral administration, and so on), a successful antipolio drug should reduce virus replication to a level that prevents transmission of the virus from host to host. The goal of this chapter is to describe the biological targets against which polio antiviral compounds are most likely to be successful.

Viruses offer a number of chemotherapeutic targets for the prevention or treatment of infection. Poliovirus is no exception and appears particularly suited for targeting antiviral drugs because it is one of the most thoroughly studied viruses.

The design of antiviral drugs against RNA viruses like poliovirus is complicated by the viruses' extreme genetic variability. Polioviruses, like all RNA viruses, are so genetically variable that they are best described as "quasi-species" (Eigen 1993; Holland et al. 1982, 1992; Domingo et al. 1988). They exist as heterogeneous mixtures of related genomes; the individual viral particles are not all genetically identical. A consensus sequence can be defined for the poliovirus genome, but an infection will actually consist of thousands of genomes, each differing slightly from the consensus. The reason for this phenomenon, which has profound biological consequences, is a high inherent error rate (about 1 nucleotide of every 10,000 is misincorporated during genome replication) combined with a lack of proofreading and editing mechanisms. High error frequency has also been documented in poliovirus replication (Crotty et al. 2000; de la Torre et al. 1990). Quasi-species present a dynamic equilibrium of many viral genotypes in which the identity of the wild type is maintained only because of strong selection against a continuously appearing spectrum of mutants. As has been apparent in the development of drugs against many RNA viruses, the existence of a pool of variants makes it likely that mutants resistant to a given drug ("escape" mutants) already exist in the population before the drug is even used (Coffin 1995).

The speed with which drug resistance will emerge is difficult to predict since it depends on the target chosen for inhibition and the circumstances in which the drug would be used. However, an ideal polio antiviral drug will have features that slow the emergence of resistant mutants. One way to minimize or avoid the rapid emergence of escape mutants is to design a drug so that resistant viral variants are much less fit than nonresistant viruses. For example, oseltamivir, a drug that inhibits influenza neuraminidase, binds to a highly conserved active site, so variants resistant to the inhibitor also have greatly reduced neuraminidase activity and replicate poorly (Carr et al. 2002). An even more sophisticated strategy is to design the drug so that resistant mutants actually interfere with nonresistant viruses. Resistant mutants with this characteristic are said to have a "dominant negative" effect. For example, a mutation resulting in a misfolded protein that binds to and interferes with the function of normally folded proteins would be likely to have such a dominant negative effect (Crowder and Kirkegaard 2005).

SYNOPSIS OF POLIOVIRUS PATHOGENESIS AND REPLICATION

Poliovirus is a highly contagious virus that belongs to the genus *Enterovirus* of the large family of *Picornaviridae* (Stanway et al. 2002). Picornaviruses have been estimated to cause an astounding 6 billion human infections per year, and they give rise to a wide array of serious, even lethal, diseases (Melnick 1996). Enteroviruses alone (about 100 serotypes) are responsible for 1 billion infections per year. Enterovirus infections, including those caused by poliovirus, are largely covert, but the vast incidence of infections translates into a large number of clinical cases.

This report is not intended as an exhaustive review of all steps in cellular poliovirus replication or pathogenesis. Some details of the interaction of the virion (an individual virus particle) with the receptor CD155, of polyprotein synthesis and processing, and genome replication will be provided in sections below discussing drug targets. Reviews of all aspects of poliovirus replication and pathogenesis can be found in *Molecular Biology of Picornaviruses* (Semler and Wimmer 2002).

Poliovirus, the prototype of the enteroviruses, has a single-stranded genome (about 7,500 nucleotides) of plus strand polarity (that is, it serves as mRNA in the infected cell) whose nucleotide sequence has been known since 1981 (Kitamura et al. 1981; Racaniello and Baltimore 1981). The genome is protected by a rigid protein shell consisting of multiples of 4 polypeptides. There is no lipid envelope (Rossmann 2002).

On entry into a host cell, which is facilitated by the cellular receptor CD155 (also known as Pvr) (Koike et al. 1990; Mendelsohn et al. 1989), the viral genome expresses all its genetic information in the cytoplasm. Expression proceeds first by translation, which yields a polyprotein that is proteolytically cleaved by viral proteinases encoded in the polyprotein (Wimmer et al. 1993). This is followed by genome replication, encapsidation, and release from infected cells (Fig. 1) (Paul 2002; Agol 2002). Starting with genome RNA, the entire replication cycle can be reproduced in a cell-free extract (Molla et al. 1991).

Cytoplasmic replication of poliovirus is stringently dependent upon membranous structures that the virus builds from cellular membranes during the first phase of the infectious cycle. The poliovirus proteins 2BC and $2C^{ATPase}$, mapping to the center of the viral genome, are predominantly responsible for the rearrangement of cellular vesicles to form numerous new vesicles (Egger et al. 2002) and autophagosomes (Jackson et al. 2005) that are the sites of genome replication.

Individual steps of the replication cycle at the cellular level have been studied in great detail, which will aid in the identification of targets for poliovirus antiviral drugs. Currently, the forerunners are small molecules that interfere with the entry of the virion into the host cell (drugs that insert themselves into the capsid) and small molecules that inhibit the action of the virus-encoded proteinase $3C^{pro}$. Likewise, the RNA-dependent RNA polymerase $3D^{pol}$ is an attractive target for chemotherapeutic intervention.

Pathogenesis

In contrast with cellular replication, our knowledge of the mechanism of poliovirus pathogenesis is limited. Infection occurs by the oral-fecal route (Minor 1997; Bodian and Horstman 1965; Sabin 1956; Bodian 1955). As

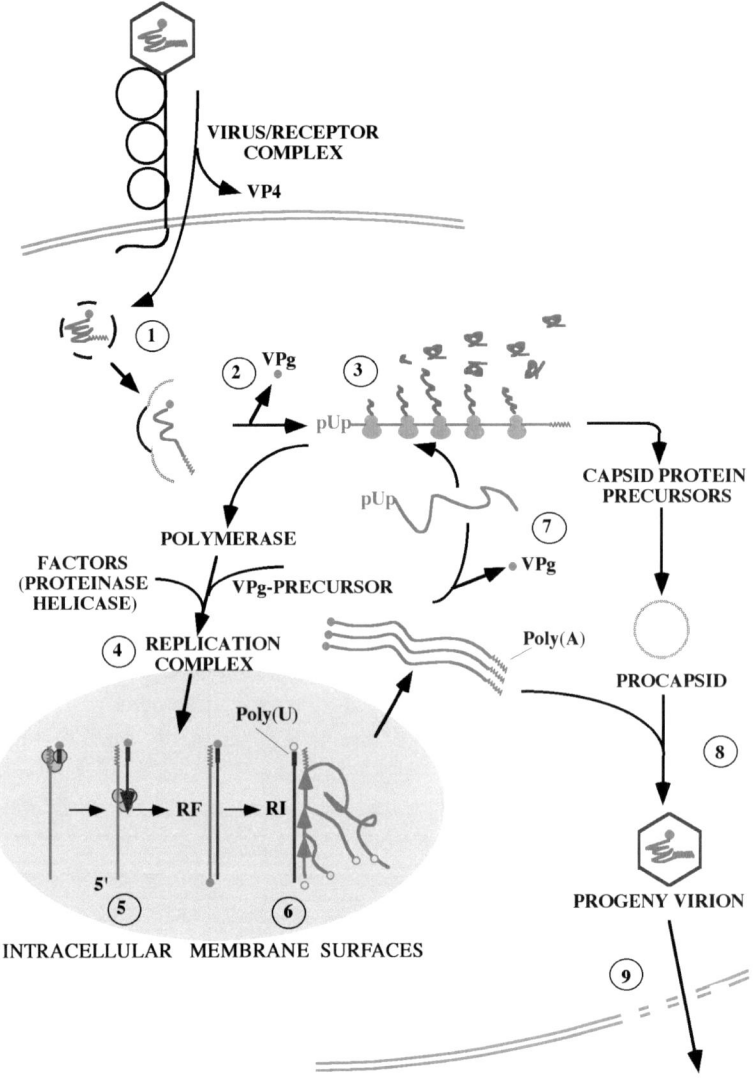

FIGURE 1 Schematic representation of the cellular replication cycle of poliovirus. (1) After binding to the receptor CD155, the virion is transported into the cell and uncoated. (2) The 5'-terminal VPg covalently-attached protein is thought to be cleaved from the incoming genome by a cellular enzyme after which (3) the RNA is translated end-to-end into a polyprotein. The latter is subsequently processed into numerous functional proteins (see Fig. 3). (4) A membrane-associated replication complex is being formed by viral and cellular proteins (possibly involving a helicase). (5) The plus

caption continues

an enteric virus, poliovirus replicates in the gastrointestinal (GI) tract for 3 to 4 weeks, but occasionally for several months (Alexander et al. 1997; Horstmann et al. 1946). Rarely, at rates of 10^{-3} to 10^{-2}, the virus invades the central nervous system (CNS) to target predominantly motor neurons, and this invasion leads to paralysis or death (Racaniello 2001; Mueller et al. 2005; Minor 1997; Nathanson and Martin 1979). Why motor neurons are targeted by poliovirus is not understood.

There is another significant gap in our knowledge of poliovirus pathogenesis. Although there is little doubt that the virus replicates in sites of the GI tract—most likely in secondary lymphatic tissues, such as tonsils and Peyer's patches (Nathanson 2005; Horie et al. 1994; Wenner et al. 1959; Bodian 1955; Sabin 1956; Bodian 1952; Sabin and Ward 1941; Fairbrother and Hurst 1930)—the nature of the cells that support poliovirus proliferation in the GI-associated lymphoid tissues (GALT) or elsewhere remains obscure. The lack of detailed understanding of the sites of poliovirus replication may be an obstacle to drug development in that those sites cannot currently be specifically targeted for monitoring drug activity.

TARGETS FOR POLIO ANTIVIRALS

A. Capsid-Binding Agents

The poliovirus capsid is an icosahedron consisting of 60 copies each of capsid polypeptides VP1, VP3, VP2, and VP4 (Filman et al. 1989; Hogle et al. 1985). A unit of these four capsid polypeptides first assembles to form a "protomer" (VP1, VP3, and VP0, the latter being the precursor of VP2 and VP4); five protomers then form a pentamer, and 12 pentamers assemble into the viral procapsid that finally undergoes the maturation cleavage of VP0 to VP2 and VP4 on entry of the genome. A deep "canyon" surrounds the apex of each pentamer of the virus; at each of the 60 protomer-protomer interfaces there is a small hydrophobic pocket at the canyon floor (Fig. 2). This pocket is a promising target of antipoliovirus drugs (Rossmann 2002).

---

stranded genome RNA is transcribed into a minus strand under formation of a double-stranded "replicative form" (RF). (6) Minus strands then function as template for the synthesis of plus strands. (7) Newly synthesized plus stranded RNA has the choice of re-entering genome replication (4), serving as mRNA in translation (7), or associating with procapsids (8) to form mature virions that are released from the decaying cell (9). The nucleus is not involved in the replicative cycle. For details, see (Semler and Wimmer 2002).

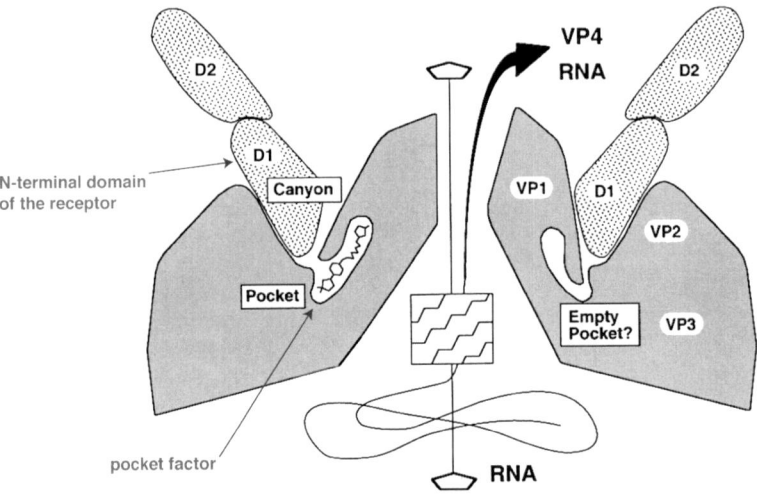

FIGURE 2 Proposed binding of an immunoglobulin-like receptor into the virion canyon followed by capsid rearrangement and genome release. Shown is the apical region of the virion with the prominent canyon at the 5-fold axis. The pocket at the canyon bottom is normally filled with a small hydrophobic compound that is thought to be released upon uncoating. In this figure, the N-terminal domain of the receptor (here ICAM-1, the receptor for the majority of rhinoviruses) enters the canyon, intruding almost down to the canyon floor. In the binding of poliovirus to CD155, the interaction between the N-terminal receptor domain and virion is largely restricted to the canyon rim. Both ICAM-1 and CD155 consist of 5 and 3 immunoglobulin-related domains, respectively, referred to as D1 (N-terminal), D2, D3, etc. The interaction between receptor and canyon destabilizes the virion, allowing release of the small capsid polypeptides VP4 and the genome (right side of the scheme). If the natural pocket factor is replaced by hydrophobic compounds that lodge more stably in the pocket (for example, binding of the WIN51711 compound into the poliovirus pocket), the rearrangement and uncoating processes are inhibited. (Modified from Rossmann et al. 2000.)

Normally, a small hydrophobic compound (such as sphingosine or other cellular components) that allows flexibility of the capsid polypeptides occupies the small canyon pocket. Drug candidates that replace the hydrophobic compound in the pocket stabilize the virion in such a way that uncoating is inhibited (Rossmann et al. 2000; Rossmann 2002; Joseph-McCarthy et al. 2001). Insertion of the drug is thought to interfere with the capsid polypeptide rearrangements necessary for genome release.

Several pharmaceutical companies have identified and studied a considerable number of hydrophobic capsid-binding compounds. The best known is pleconaril (WIN63843), a drug that was developed by Sterling Winthrop with great promise for the treatment of enteroviral and rhinoviral infections. Pleconaril, however, was not licensed by the Food and Drug Administration (FDA) because of undesirable side effects when it was administered in combination with other medications (i.e., oral contraceptives). Nevertheless, because of the wealth of data gathered over the last 20 years, small molecules with the propensity for occupying the hydrophobic canyon pocket are strong candidates for the development of an anti-poliovirus drug. A number of candidates identified during the development of pleconaril may have more activity against poliovirus than against rhinoviruses. Indeed, several potential candidates currently under investigation by ViroDefense, Inc. are further discussed in Chapter 4.

B. Drugs Directed Against Non-Structural Proteins

It is reasonable to choose proteins encoded in the non-structural region of the genome as targets for anti-poliovirus drugs. However, poliovirus can undergo genetic recombination (Wimmer et al. 1993; Romanova et al. 1980; Hirst 1962) as a second mechanism for generating drug resistance and this ability is highly relevant to the use of antiviral medications in poliovirus eradication. In a cell infected with a single serotype, recombinants are formed with frequencies as high as 10^{-4} (Kirkegaard and Baltimore 1986). Since homologous recombination is the mechanism of genome exchange(s) (Kirkegaard and Baltimore 1986) lower frequencies of recombination (10^{-5} to 10^{-6}) are observed amongst different polioviruses serotypes (Tolskaya et al. 1983). Kew and his colleagues have recently discovered that circulating vaccine-derived polioviruses (cVDPVs), which have caused yearly outbreaks of poliomyelitis since 2001 (see Table 1), are predominantly recombinants between polioviruses and non-human enteroviruses (Kew et al. 2005, 2002). Candidates of the non-human enteroviruses are those coxsackie viruses (C-CAV) (Kew et al. 2002) that are in the same cluster as poliovirus (Stanway et al. 2002). Recombination between poliovirus, type 1 (Mahoney) [or poliovirus, type 1 (Sabin)] and C-CAV type 20 can be readily demonstrated to occur in tissue culture cells at a frequency of 10^{-6} (Ping et al. unpublished results). Since cross-over occurs predominantly near the middle of the genomes, the cVDPV recombinants, which have acquired coding sequences of nonstructural proteins of C-CAVs, may be resistant to drugs directed at the poliovirus encoded enzymes (e.g., proteinases or RNA polymerase). Therefore, if these targets are chosen for antipoliovirus drug development, it may be necessary for these drugs to be broadly reactive, including having activity against polypeptides of the C-cluster coxsackie viruses.

1. Inhibitors of the Virus-Encoded Proteinases

Poliovirus expresses its entire protein-related genetic information as a single polypeptide, the polyprotein (Baltimore et al. 1969). This polyprotein is proteolytically processed by two viral proteinases, $3C^{pro}/3CD^{pro}$ (Ypma-Wong et al. 1988; Svitkin et al. 1979) and $2A^{pro}$ (Skern et al. 2002; Toyoda et al. 1986) into some 29 polypeptides, of which some are relatively stable precursor molecules that have essential functions in replication (Fig. 3) (Leong et al. 2002). As is common in viral replication, virus-encoded polypeptides often have more than one essential function and that is true also for the viral proteinases, $3C^{pro}/3CD^{pro}$ and $2A^{pro}$.

Proteinases $3C/3CD^{pro}$

The relatively stable processing intermediate $3CD^{pro}$ is not only a proteinase but also an RNA-binding protein essential for genome replication. Once cleaved, $3CD^{pro}$ yields the smaller proteinase $3C^{pro}$ and the viral RNA polymerase $3D^{pol}$. Both $3C^{pro}$ and $3CD^{pro}$ can cleave at glutamine-glycine bonds, the scissile peptide bond in poliovirus polyprotein processing (Skern et al. 2002; Nicklin et al. 1988); however, only $3CD^{pro}$ can efficiently cleave the capsid precursor P1 (Ypma-Wong et al. 1988). Antiviral agents that target these proteinases, however, are likely to interfere with both $3C^{pro}$ and

---

FIGURE 3 Genome organization of poliovirus and proteolytic processing of the polyprotein. (A) Schematic representation of the genome. Starting with the 5'-terminal genome-linked protein VPg, the 5' non-translated region is divided into cloverleaf, a structure essential for genome replication, and IRES, a structure essential for internal initiation of protein synthesis. The open square indicates the polyprotein divided into polypeptides, which are end products of cleavage. The 3' non-translated region consists of two stem-loop structures and poly(A) (Agol 2002). (B) Pathway of proteolytic cleavages by two virus-encoded proteinases $2A^{pro}$ (cleavage at open diamond) and $3C/3CD^{pro}$ (cleavages at open triangles) (Leong et al. 2002). *** Indicates rapid cleavages; * slow cleavages, the kinetics determined predominantly by the sequence at the scissile bond (Nicklin et al. 1988; Hellen et al. 1991). Precursor proteins such as 2BC and $3CD^{pro}$ fulfill important functions in the replication cycle (see text). The mechanism of the maturation cleavage (filled triangle) is not understood. (FIGURE 3 *on next page*.)

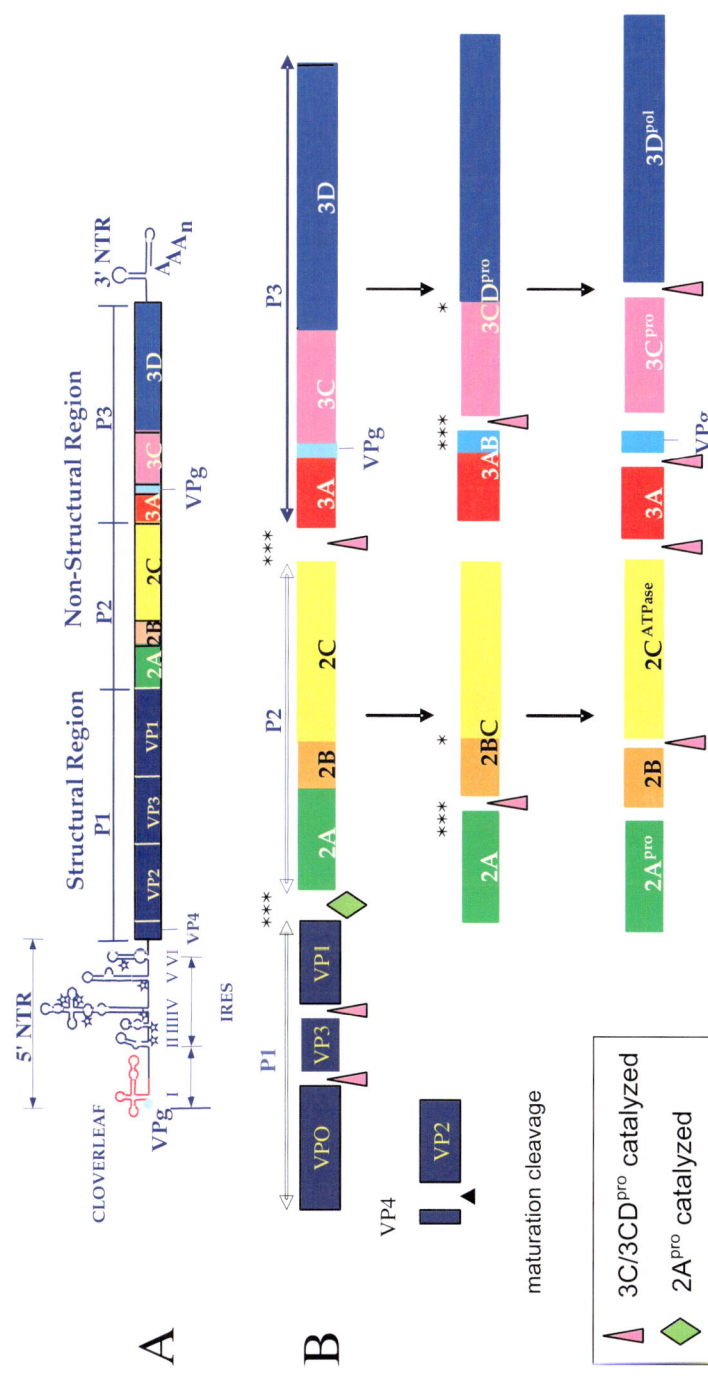

FIGURE 3 Caption on previous page.

3CD^{pro} functions. The high-resolution crystal structure of poliovirus 3C^{pro} has been solved which is valuable for drug development targeted at the enzyme (Mosimann et al. 1997). It is a cysteine proteinase with a serine proteinase fold and structural similarities to chymotrypsin. Available evidence suggests that all 3C^{pro} proteinases of enteroviruses and rhinoviruses exhibit a highly conserved active site (Binford et al. 2005). 3C/3CD^{pro} proteinase inhibitors have been shown to be active against many enteroviruses and rhinoviruses, which not only may be a prerequisite of drugs directed at these enzymes (because of the recombinant cVDPVs discussed above) but also may be an incentive for investment by the commercial sector (Patick et al. 1999). Development spearheaded by Pfizer has led to human rhinovirus type 2 (HRV2) 3C^{pro} proteinase inhibitors. The most advanced compounds include rupintrivir (Phase II trials), an intranasally administered compound, and compound 1 (Phase I), an orally bioavailable compound. Inhibition of poliovirus by rupintrivir has not been tested but is predicted based on strong homology between the 3C protease of poliovirus and other picornaviruses.

As an RNA-binding protein, 3CD^{pro}, with poly(rC) binding protein (PCBP), forms a stable ribonucleoprotein complex with the cloverleaf structure at the 5' end of the genome that is essential for genome replication (Parsley et al. 1997; Andino et al. 1990). 3CD^{pro} is also a cofactor in the formation of a ribonucleoprotein complex between the RNA polymerase 3D^{pol}, a small viral protein VPg, and a cis-acting replication element (*cre* stem loop) mapping to the coding region of 2C^{ATPase}. This complex functions in the initiation of viral RNA synthesis (Yang et al. 2004; Paul et al. 2000). Addition of purified 3CD^{pro} to the cell-free replication system (Molla et al. 1991) stimulates virion synthesis 100-fold, an observation suggesting the essential role of this viral protein in poliovirus proliferation (Franco et al. 2005).

Proteinase 2A^{pro}

Whereas 3C/3CD^{pro} catalyze the majority of proteolytic cleavages of the polyprotein, 2A^{pro} catalyzes only one essential cleavage: that between the capsid precursor and the nonstructural proteins (Fig. 3) (Toyoda et al. 1986). 2A^{pro}, however, is also involved in genome replication by an unknown mechanism (Molla et al. 1993). The crystal structure of poliovirus 2A^{pro} is not known, but it is probably closely related to the known structure of HRV2 2A^{pro}. The crystal structure of HRV2 2A^{pro}, like that of

3C^{pro}, has also revealed a cysteine proteinase with a serine proteinase fold (Petersen et al. 1999). Anti-2A inhibitors are likely to display the additional advantage of suppressing genetic reversion because of the intracellular dominance of uncleaved capsid-2A precursors, inasmuch as it has recently been shown that unprocessed VP1-2A precursors have a dominant negative effect on capsid formation (Crowder and Kirkegaard 2005).

3C/3CD^{pro} and 2A^{pro} also catalyze proteolytic degradation of numerous cellular proteins, and this contributes to rapid cell death (Weidman et al. 2003; Kuechler et al. 2002). Inhibition of the poliovirus proteinases, therefore, probably would not only prevent viral replication but also have a positive effect on the survival of the infected cell.

Poliovirus proteinases are excellent substrates for drug development because they are essential for key stages in the replication cycle. Moreover, they exhibit minimal similarity to known mammalian enzymes. Indeed, proteases as targets for chemotherapeutic intervention—for example against HIV—have the advantage of being well explored by pharmaceutical companies.

2. Inhibitors of the Poliovirus RNA-Dependent RNA Polymerase 3D^{pol}

Poliovirus genome replication follows a common strategy used by all single-stranded plus-strand RNA viruses; the plus-stranded genomic RNA is transcribed into minus-strand copies, which then serve as templates for progeny genomic RNA (Wimmer et al. 1993). In poliovirus replication, all newly synthesized genomes can serve as further templates for genome replication, as mRNA in translation, or as substrate for encapsidation (Paul 2002).

The synthesis of both plus-stranded and minus-stranded RNAs is catalyzed by 3D^{pol}, a strictly primer dependent polymerase (Paul 2002; Flanegan and Baltimore 1977). The primer is the uridylylated form of the small viral protein VPg (VPg-pUpU), which is synthesized by the polymerase itself. Following uridylylation, VPg-pUpU is elongated to either plus or minus stranded RNAs (Paul 2002; Paul et al. 1998).

There are potentially two approaches to targeting 3D^{pol}. First, direct inhibition of its two enzymatic functions would block several steps in genome replication, including VPg uridylylation, initiation, or elongation. Indeed, it is possible that different compounds may be identified that selectively inhibit uridylylation of VPg or elongation (polymerization) of the polynucleotide strand.

A second approach is to target the polymerase in such a way as to induce a change in error rate. As noted above, the characteristic high error rate of RNA viruses is an important factor in their ability to adapt to new environments and resist the action of drugs. There is evidence that the optimal mutation rate for RNA viruses may have a narrow range; therefore, it may be possible to inhibit virus replication by either increasing or decreasing the mutation rate (Vignuzzi et al. 2005; Pfeiffer and Kirkegaard 2005; Crotty et al. 2000). An increase in error rate should lead to lethal mutagenesis, whereas a decrease in error rate (high fidelity replication) should reduce the ability of the virus to adapt to environmental changes (see box). Some polymerase inhibitors are likely to have the additional advantage of suppressed genetic reversion due to the intracellular dominance of inhibitor-bound polymerase molecules.

The solution of the complete three-dimensional structure of poliovirus 3D^{pol} provides greater opportunities for structure-based inhibitor design (Thompson and Peersen 2004). Several companies have successfully targeted the RNA-dependent RNA polymerase of hepatitis C virus—an effort resulting in compounds that are now in clinical trials (Wu et al. 2005). Some of the drugs under development against the HCV polymerase have also shown inhibitory activity against poliovirus (Olsen et al. 2004) but whether they are viable starting compounds against poliovirus infection is not known.

Nucleoside analogues with mutagenic potential, such as ribavirin, have been identified, but additional work is necessary to establish whether they are effective antipoliovirus drugs. It is recommended that screening of libraries be undertaken to identify nonnucleoside compounds that inhibit polymerase function both by interfering with replication and by altering the mutation rate of poliovirus.

C. Other Possible Targets for Antiviral Development

1. *In Addition to the Capsid-Binding, Proteinase, and Polymerase Targets Described Above, the Following Poliovirus Components Could Be Promising Targets for Antiviral Drugs:*

    a. 2C is an ATPase that is crucial for viral replication (Pfister and Wimmer 1999). High-throughput assays to screen for inhibition of its activity could be readily designed.

Genetic Diversity May Contribute to Poliovirus Pathogenesis

Results of recent studies (Vignuzzi et al. 2005; Pfeiffer and Kirkegaard 2005) that were designed to test key postulates of the quasispecies theory suggest that population diversity may have a role in poliovirus pathogenesis, specifically in the ability of the virus to spread to the central nervous system (CNS). Although wild-type virus can access and replicate in the CNS, a high fidelity virus was restricted from systemic spread. The results show that the diversity of the quasispecies itself may be a critical determinant of pathogenesis. Notably, treatment of the high fidelity viruses with mutagenic nucleoside analogues, which restored genomic diversity, was shown also to restore the ability to spread to the CNS (Vignuzzi et al. 2005). Furthermore, the study indicated that there is positive interaction between variants in the quasispecies: one mutant may allow other mutants to enter the brain. Thus, complexity of the viral quasispecies enables the virus population to spread systemically and to access the CNS, perhaps because of complementary functions of different subpopulations that facilitate adaptation to new environments. Some variants in the population may facilitate the colonization of the gut, another set of mutants may serve as immunological decoys that trick the immune system, and yet another may facilitate crossing the blood-brain barrier. Those findings have important consequences for antiviral therapeutic strategies. Nucleoside-based mutagens, such as the anti-HIV drug zidovudine (AZT), take advantage of the RNA polymerases' high error rate to induce the virus to incorporate faulty nucleosides as it replicates. One way that viruses acquire resistance to nucleoside-based mutagens is by having mutations that improve the fidelity of their RNA polymerases. The results of the experiments suggest that a resistant poliovirus with a high fidelity polymerase would lose the ability to spread to the CNS.

---

b. RNA structures, such as the noncoding regions and the cis acting replication element (*cre*) are crucial for genome replication and might be excellent targets.

c. 3A, a small protein required for RNA replication, is the target for enviroxime, a promising compound for further characterization.

2. Non-Small Molecule Based Antiviral Strategies

The antiviral strategies described above call for the development of small molecules that would bind to, block, or inhibit the various poliovirus targets. Pharmaceutical companies and regulatory institutions have experience with small-molecule development, testing, and regulation, and these approaches are most likely to be successful in the short term. However, a number of novel therapeutic approaches could be quickly adapted for the treatment of poliovirus if they are successfully developed for the treatment of other diseases.

siRNA mediated inhibition of poliovirus replication

Small interfering RNAs (siRNAs) are small strands of RNA, 21-23 nucleotides long, that are designed to bind to the complementary portion of a target messenger RNA and thereby signal the cell that the target RNA should be degraded (Yeung et al. 2005). The attractiveness of such a strategy against RNA viruses is clear: siRNAs could be used to induce infected cells to digest the viral RNA and halt replication. siRNA reagents are being developed by several companies (Anylan, Isis, and SiRNA) to treat a variety of human diseases, especially cancer. The problem of delivering the siRNAs in sufficient quantity to the appropriate target cells has not been solved. Several siRNA targets in poliovirus genomes have been identified (Gitlin et al. 2002). Such a strategy has the advantage of targeting several sequences simultaneously, thus making it difficult for the virus to acquire resistance. If the current problems with delivery in humans were resolved, siRNA might be a viable alternative for prophylaxis of and therapy for poliovirus infections.

Morpholinos

Morpholinos are similar to siRNAs in that they are short strands of nucleic acid designed to bind to specific complementary stretches on target RNA (Arora et al. 2004). Morpholinos differ from siRNAs in having backbones that are not the usual sugars and phosphates found in natural nucleic acids and therefore are immune to DNase degradation by cellular enzymes. Their binding blocks the activity of the target RNA, and this makes them ideal as therapeutic agents against RNA viruses if the capability to deliver the morpholinos to target cells in sufficient quantity can be developed.

Protective antibodies

The administration of hyperimmune globulin can provide immediate protective immunity against infectious agents and toxins. The development of antibodies as therapeutic agents has been under way since the 1980s. Early results of using antibodies made by infecting mice were somewhat disappointing. Recent results with humanized monoclonal antibodies (murine antibodies engineered to resemble human antibodies) are more encouraging, and more than 10 monoclonal antibodies have been licensed (Reichert 2001). Results of experiments in the early 1950s indicated that passive immunization could prevent poliomyelitis (Rinaldo 2005) and suggested that passive administration of antipoliovirus antibodies could be an attractive approach if the technology improves and costs fall.

BASIC RESEARCH NEEDS

Many of the virus-specific processes in poliovirus proliferation offer targets for chemotherapeutic intervention. Among them, the capsid and the viral proteinase $3C^{pro}/3CD^{pro}$ have been subject to extensive studies with the specific aim of generating antiviral drugs. Those efforts, however, were directed predominantly at nonpolio enteroviruses and the related human rhinoviruses. The close genetic and biochemical kinship of human enteroviruses and rhinoviruses suggests that compounds developed previously against these picornaviruses might serve as superb immediate candidates for the development of antipoliovirus agents.

In spite of a wealth of information related to intracellular poliovirus replication, the details of individual steps (such as uptake of virus into the cell, regulation of polyprotein processing, the switch from translation to genome synthesis, regulation of plus-strand and minus-strand synthesis, rearrangement of cellular organelles, and encapsidation and virus maturation) are obscure. Similarly, the sites of replication in the GI tract after oral infection and the mechanisms by which infection progresses to poliomyelitis remain largely unknown. More detailed understanding of these processes would probably identify additional targets. The successful development of polio antiviral drugs will rely heavily on continuous strong support of poliovirus research.

4

Development of Antiviral Drugs
for Poliovirus

CHAPTER 2 OF THIS REPORT DELINEATED the importance of an effective antiviral drug in ensuring the eventual success of the polio eradication program. Chapter 3 identified a number of poliovirus targets at which drugs might be aimed. The goal of this chapter is to discuss the steps that a potential antiviral drug will have to pass through to be successful.

The first step is to identify what the drug must do and how it will be used, to write a "package insert," as it were, for the drug before it even exists. In Chapter 2, the committee recommended that an antiviral drug be developed to be used principally as a prophylactic in the event of a poliomyelitis outbreak, with the capability of both preventing infection and preventing spread from those already infected. It identified a number of additional requirements:

- Low cost
- Extreme safety
- Oral administration
- Once, or at most twice, daily dosing
- Stability

From the point of view of development, some of those requirements merit early attention. First, it is important to develop drugs that have low effective concentration (EC)—that is, are efficacious at very low plasma concentrations so that they can be administered in small doses. This will both help to keep the cost low and will be likely to reduce safety risks. EC_{50} is defined as the drug concentration that inhibits 50% of virus replication; EC_{90} is the dose that provokes a response that is 90% of the maximum. The EC_{50} and EC_{90} should be in the low nanogram range. In addition to showing substantial antiviral activity, a molecule suitable for development must be amenable to large-scale, cost-effective synthesis. Difficulties in synthesis will be directly reflected in higher costs.

Chapter 2 further suggested that the most likely application of a polio antiviral drug would be in combination with inactivated poliovirus vaccine. If ring prophylaxis with a medication and vaccine is expected, the number of people requiring treatment would be exceedingly large and require large quantities of medication.

Successful development of an antiviral drug to prevent poliovirus transmission will require simultaneous attention to two challenges: active agents must be identified and optimized, and how the agent will be used must be carefully defined, because this will determine how it will be tested, regulated, and administered.

POTENTIAL HURDLES TO ADDRESS AT THE OUTSET

At the outset of a program designed to develop drugs to treat poliovirus infections, potential hurdles should be identified. Development of medications for therapy of poliovirus infections historically has not attracted support from the pharmaceutical industry. The committee does not envision industry support of development costs, so a fundamental question that needs to be resolved is: Who will fund the development of these medications? As clinical trials are envisioned, a parallel question will be: Who will hold the investigational new drug application? Those two questions should be addressed at the outset of any initiative. A credible clinical development plan that ensures the project could proceed beyond preclinical proof of concept will be critical to attract support for such a program. Because it is envisioned that these drugs will be used globally, it would be helpful to establish an international collaboration of responsible individuals, including regulatory authorities, at the outset of the program.

IDENTIFYING AND OPTIMIZING POTENTIAL POLIO ANTIVIRAL DRUGS

Exploitation of Existing Leads

Development of a polio antiviral drug can build on experience with other antiviral drugs. Furthermore, given that on average it takes $802 million and 10 to 15 years from start to finish to bring a drug to market (Frank 2003), the exploitation of existing, advanced leads may be crucial to this potential poliovirus antiviral effort (especially considering possible time constraints related to the eradication effort). The average cost and time stated above reflects many attempts and failures (and much basic research) for many diverse targets and indications. For poliovirus, the utilization of existing, advanced leads could be expected to reduce significantly the time and cost of development. A number of leads exist at various stages of advancement for poliovirus targets including the capsid, $3C^{pro}$ proteinase, and to some extent $2A^{pro}$ proteinase and the RNA polymerase $3D^{pol}$. Members of the picornavirus family—consisting of the rhinoviruses, hepatitis A, and a large number of potentially dangerous enteroviruses, including polioviruses 1, 2, and 3—are common but cause widely divergent clinical illness. Historically, efforts have focused on the development of antiviral therapeutics to treat rhinovirus infections, such as the common cold. Those efforts led to the elegant studies of structure-based activity of capsid-binding inhibitors, of which pleconaril is the best known example. Pleconaril was evaluated through Phase 3 clinical trials for treatment of the common cold. It had a modest degree of efficacy in the treatment of rhinoviral disease, but licensure by the Food and Drug Administration (FDA), as recommended by an advisory committee, was denied because of the induction of hepatic cytochrome enzymes that altered the metabolism of birth control pills and resulted in intramenstrual bleeding. As a consequence, the drug was abandoned for systemic administration.

Pleconaril has no significant activity against polioviruses. However, ViroDefense, Inc. has identified a member of the capsid-binding inhibitor class, V-037, that has significant *in vitro* activity against human poliovirus type 1 (Collett 2005). We present some of the details of the behavior of this specific molecule simply as an example of an existing lead in this target class for which a significant amount of development has already occurred. For human poliovirus type 1, *in vitro* cell culture activity at an EC_{90} was identified as less than 0.02 μM. V-037 is less active against human polioviruses type 2 and 3. The strains tested *in vitro* were constituents of the oral polio vaccine. V-037 is also less active against wild-type polioviruses. Preclinical assessments demonstrate that it is Ames test-negative and chromosome-aberration negative. Given orally, it is bioavailable in a murine model and achieves concentrations in the central nervous system that are four to six times the plasma concentration. These levels were not corrected for protein-binding and thus do not necessarily reflect the level of free, or unbound drug. However, while protein binding is a fundamental concern in drug development, its application to the development of antiviral drugs is not well established. *In vitro* studies are performed using human blood, but their translation to probability of success in the clinic has not been established. For example, the highly protein bound bromovinyl arabinosyl uracil proved efficacious in the treatment of herpes zoster albeit it was not licensed for other reasons (Gnann et al. 1998). After cerebral inoculation in a murine model of poliovirus type 2, 100% of mice survived. The no-effect doses (the dose at which no toxicity is seen) were 100 mg/kg in the mouse and 750 mg/kg in the dog. At the highest doses, an engorged liver was observed. The latter finding is important because the lead molecule of this class, pleconaril, induced hepatic cytochrome activity and the finding may be a signal of potential toxicity. Other chemically distinct poliovirus capsid-binding ligands have been identified by ViroDefense and others (Andries et al. 1992, 1990), however, and would probably have different properties.

An enzyme essential to rhinovirus replication, 3C[pro] proteinase, provided another logical target for the development of antipicornaviral therapeutics. That enzyme and its precursor polypeptide 3CD[pro] are responsible for proteolytic cleavage steps that are conserved across all entero- and rhinoviruses. A drug candidate, rupintrivir, was studied through Phase 1B/2 clinical trials with human rhinovirus infections but failed to demonstrate significant clinical activity. As a consequence, this lead molecule was abandoned. A second generation 3C[pro] proteinase inhibitor has been developed by Pfizer and appears to have a pharmacokinetic profile that is satisfactory for the treatment of picornavirus infections; however, its activity against polioviruses has not been evaluated (Patick et al. 2005).

Existing capsid-binding and 3C[pro] proteinase inhibitors are potential therapeutic leads in the development of therapies for poliovirus infections that already exist. The prior investigation of these two biological targets provides a well-established platform upon which therapeutics for polioviruses could be developed. In fact, the parallel development of two classes of molecules with different mechanisms of action for the treatment of poliovirus infections is both indicated and desirable, as described below.

Identifying Leads by Screening Libraries of Molecules

Large libraries of molecules exist that could be screened against replication of polioviruses. Such libraries are available through the National Institutes of Health (the National Institute of Allergy and Infectious Disease [NIAID] and the National Cancer Institute [NCI]), the Southern Research Institute (Birmingham, AL), the pharmaceutical industry, and small biotechnology firms. A coordinated effort should be instituted to collect representative molecules of different classes for screening. In addition, target-focused libraries of known picornavirus capsid-binding and $3C^{pro}$ proteinase inhibitors and other similar compounds (identified through substructure and similarity searches) could be assembled and screened. The initial screening assays will probably involve live viruses and focus on plaque reduction. As screening efforts are developed, serious consideration should be given to which live virus strains should be used to demonstrate efficacy. Both vaccine-derived and wild-type polioviruses should be included. Initial assays can use whole virus replication with a plaque-reduction format. Ultimately, however, higher throughput assays should be developed to expedite the screening. Such high-throughput assays have been developed through sponsorship by the NIAID for other emerging infections, including West Nile virus and SARS coronavirus. Before the development of a suitable high-throughput assay, or if such an assay remains elusive, large libraries (up to millions of compounds) can be screened by computer analysis for binders to targets with known three-dimensional molecular structures (such as the poliovirus capsid or the $3C^{pro}$ proteinase), and relatively small numbers of molecules can be selected for experimental testing. Even if the three-dimensional structure of a target does not exist or the exact target is unknown, for any validated ligand (or series of ligands) it should be possible to screen large virtual libraries to identify other small molecules for testing that have overall shape and pharmacophore features similar to those of the query molecule.

As with other existing inhibitors, once molecules have been demonstrated to inhibit poliovirus replication in *in vitro* assays, mechanism-of-action studies should be initiated promptly. As a component of those studies, there should be attempts to develop resistant viruses. Such studies will further clarify the mechanism of action of these compounds and lead to the synthesis of second and third generation molecules. For advanced leads, selective indexes (such as efficacy and toxicity) should be determined.

As an example of a possible screening paradigm, the important role that FDA's Division of Antiviral Therapy played in identifying potential molecules to screen for anti-SARS activity should be considered. At the time of the SARS epidemic, FDA formally put out a request to industry and academic sources to supply compounds for testing that had some expected likelihood of being active against the therapeutic target. A number of companies participated in the effort. With the availability of known inhibitors and three-dimensional structures of at least two potential targets for poliovirus—the capsid and $3C^{pro}$ proteinase—a collaboration with FDA could lead to the identification of companies that have potential lead molecules.

The appropriateness of laboratory facilities to perform *in vitro* susceptibility testing and animal model studies also needs to be considered. With the imminent global cessation of polio immunization, the potential biological threat of an accidental or deliberate exposure of susceptible individuals to poliovirus should be recognized. Therefore, biocontainment laboratories of an appropriate level will have to be used.

Finally, a source of support for the screening of libraries should be identified at the outset of the endeavor. Historically, NIAID, through its Division of Microbiology and Infectious Diseases (Division of Virology), has initiated contracts for screening of antiviral drugs. Negotiations with NIAID should be entertained. Alternative sources of support from public and private foundations should also be considered.

Optimization of Lead Molecules

Medicinal chemistry is a fundamental component of any drug development program. Once lead molecules for potential poliovirus antiviral drugs have been identified, a medicinal chemistry program will need to be initiated to refine the molecules to optimize inhibitory properties. Contract medicinal chemistry companies (of which there are many with substantial expertise in the United States and abroad) could be employed to optimize lead molecules further. Fundamental to that effort will be structure-activity-based chemistry and the determination of structure-activity relationships among the active molecules. Given that three-dimensional x-ray crystal structures are available for both capsid-binding and $3C^{pro}$ proteinase inhibitors bound to their targets (Lentz et al. 1997; Hiremath et al. 1995,

1997; Grant et al. 1994), structure-based drug design approaches could be applied to expedite further development of lead molecules for these targets.

Criteria in the ongoing evaluation of molecules for development as drugs would include the ease and scalability of the synthetic route for a candidate drug. The "cost of goods" and complexity of manufacturing of any molecule as a medication will be directly reflected in its cost per dose. Manufacturing cost will be important in the development of any drug to treat poliovirus infections. In addition, the shelf life of the molecule will be important, given that it would probably be a component of the medical repository in place in the event of an outbreak of poliovirus infection. Finally, although the ability of any such molecule to cross the blood-brain barrier would be advantageous because it could potentially also be used to treat the symptoms of a neuropathic poliovirus infection, it is not a requirement, inasmuch as the drug will be developed primarily as a means of preventing the spread of infection.

The resistance profile of these molecules should be evaluated in depth early in development. As noted above, such knowledge can result in second and third generations of molecules that have a greater propensity to slow the emergence of resistance in addition to other improved characteristics.

As lead molecules are modified, the cost of synthesis, their stability and their propensity to elicit resistance will need to be kept in mind.

CLINICAL DEVELOPMENT

At the outset of polio antiviral drug development, the clinical development pathway should be defined. A key component in the development of potential therapeutic molecules will be a detailed consideration of whether vaccine-challenge studies or transmission studies can be performed. If efficacy studies cannot be readily performed in humans, the use of the FDA "Animal Rule" will need to be considered and discussed with the agency. The Animal Rule requires that an animal model system reflect human infection. At the present it is unclear if the FDA would be willing to license a therapeutic directed against polio utilizing the Animal Rule; the agency's position on this matter has not yet been sought. Should the Animal Rule be adopted, three models could be considered. The first employs CD155 expressing transgenic mice. The second utilizes the humanized mouse model. Both of these models require validation. In addition, classically, the monkey has been used to test virulence of polio vaccines. This model might well serve as one to test therapeutics of poliovirus interventions.

Even if the Animal Rule is not utilized, animal model studies can be of immense value in assessing how an antiviral drug could influence disease pathogenesis and should be instituted in parallel with drug development. Knowledge of metabolism, distribution, and clearance of a drug in an infected animal model are all of importance.

If the Animal Rule is not adopted, human efficacy trials will need to be considered. These could include chronic shedders (i.e., immunocompromised hosts), but these individuals are uncommon and will be difficult to define. A more realistic choice would be OPV challenge models in either naïve or distantly immunized subjects. Since OPV is used in many countries, the duration of viral shedding would be an acceptable endpoint (placebo controlled).

Clinical trials thus far envisioned might involve populations in which mass vaccination has taken place (such as India) or in challenge studies of individuals not at risk (such as IPV-immunized individuals without children). In both cases, assessment of efficacy would depend on determining the effect of therapy on shedding of virus in the stool. A key component in the performance of a clinical trial will be the effect of medication on the quantity of virus in the stool. Investigative efforts designed to determine the quantity of virus excreted in the stool will need to be reassessed, and it will be necessary to determine the average amount of virus necessary to infect a contact.

Regardless of the regulatory path taken, safety would need to be established in a significant number of human subjects. The preclinical toxicology profile should anticipate a maximal period of administration, at least in the presence of an outbreak, as identified in Chapter 2, of 6-8 weeks. It is envisioned that a therapeutic would be administered to prevent transmission of poliovirus in a community and probably be co-administered with inactivated polio vaccine. Thus, the molecule must be bio-available if given orally once or twice a day, must be safe for children as well as adults, and ideally will have a toxicity profile acceptable for populations who have an inherent medical disability (for example, malnutrition or co-infection with other infectious agents).

The clinical trial development of molecules to inhibit human poliovirus replication should be considered in a traditional format. Phase I clinical trials will include normal human volunteers to assess pharmacokinetics and safety. Initial studies will be performed in adults; however, once safety has been established in adults, pediatric pharmacokinetic studies should be initiated as promptly as possible. That point cannot be emphasized enough because it is envisioned that medication will be deployed primarily to pediatric populations. In the pharmacokinetic studies, special populations need to be considered, including pregnant women, immunocompromised hosts (such as HIV-infected people), and populations peculiar to developing countries (such as malnourished individuals).

As noted above, for the controlled clinical trial to be realistic for licensure, the "package insert" for the medication should be written before the clinical trial investigation. To that end, the primary use of a drug in treating poliovirus infections will be to prevent transmission from infected people to the susceptible individuals surrounding them. A potential secondary use would be to treat the very limited number of immunocompromised people who have been identified as chronic shedders of poliovirus. These individuals could be an ideal population for testing "the proof of principle" of the efficacy of the medication even if the ability to clear infection from them is not the ultimate goal, or measure of success, for these drugs.

Clinical trials could explore a wide array of populations, so discussions should focus on feasibility. To expedite the process, a product development committee should be established, including clinical investigators, representatives of the regulatory authorities, and representatives of industry. An important component of the product development committee will be representation of the countries involved; this is essential to ensure the ethical conduct of clinical trials.

THE IMPORTANCE OF DEVELOPING MORE THAN ONE ANTIVIRAL DRUG

The identification, optimization, and testing of drugs for the treatment of poliovirus infections is a complex process that is inherently unpredictable. Any potential lead could be proved unsuitable at any stage of the process. Furthermore, the infidelity of poliovirus replication potentially could lead to the emergence of viruses that are resistant to any individual therapeutic approach. Thus, simultaneous development of more than one drug, ideally substances that have alternative mechanisms of action, is the most prudent approach to a drug development campaign. Advanced leads that act against two targets—capsid-binding agents and 3C^{pro} inhibitors— are already identified and may therefore be most likely to yield success as a first approach.

Longer-term opportunities for the development of therapies directed against poliovirus infections require fundamental research on known critical components in their replication cycle, many of which were identified in Chapter 2. The development of any of these targets would probably result in selective and specific inhibitors of viral replication but would require a long-term investment of 10-15 years. Thus, as an immediate strategy for the prevention of poliovirus transmission, those targets are less feasible than the near-term projects. However, continued basic research on poliovirus and continued monitoring of non-small-molecule approaches to antiviral treatment would constitute a wise investment and would mean that additional candidate molecules and antiviral approaches would be in the development pipeline in case the early approaches prove disappointing.

TIMELINES AND COSTS

One issue that deserves careful consideration is whether a polio antiviral drug can be developed in time to contribute to the global eradication program. If current plans are followed, OPV will continue to be used for up to 6 years after the last wild poliovirus infection is detected. This 6-year period is envisaged as being composed of two 3-year intervals. When 3 years have passed since detection of the last known case of wild polio infection, OPV use will be simultaneously ceased worldwide. During the following 3 years, plans call for intensive surveillance and rapid response to any cVDPV outbreak with monovalent OPV. As discussed in Chapter 2, the committee does not expect a polio antiviral drug to have great utility if the means of outbreak control is a live vaccine. Therefore, even under the most optimistic scenario, if the last case of wild poliovirus were to occur this year, it will be at least 6 years before the need for an antiviral might become apparent. If, as currently expected, it will be at least another year before wild poliovirus transmission can be interrupted in Nigeria, the time available for antiviral development stretches to 7-8 years.

The development of timelines for medications to treat poliovirus infections can be summarized briefly. Progress has already been achieved with ViroDefense's V-037, but it remains to be determined whether it is fully optimized and free of toxicity for administration to large numbers of people. Optimization to achieve an acceptable risk:benefit ratio will be essential. Almost certainly, Pfizer's Compound 1 will require further optimization; however, that too remains to be determined and obviously will depend on its untested activity *in vitro* against poliovirus replication. All other targets require further development, which will require a substantial investment of time and effort, probably at least a decade.

ViroDefense estimates that preclinical toxicology and good manufacturing practices (GMP) production of V-037 will take about 18 months. Clinical trials from Phase I through Phase III will require at least 3-4 years. Depending on the rapidity with which studies can be performed in the adult population, overlapping safety studies in children will need to be performed; however, a timeline for these studies cannot yet be assessed. Thus, if development were to proceed immediately, the ViroDefense compound could be ready in less than 6 years, with Compound 1 perhaps taking slightly longer. The committee recognizes that these are estimates and should be more carefully assessed before proceeding, but these estimates suggest that the timelines for drug development and the currently planned eradication program are not necessarily incompatible.

The development of "near-term" molecules would not only probably be faster, but will be less expensive than that of "long-term" molecules that require the identification of new targets. The committee found it difficult to assign costs because of distinct differences in the near versus long term potential development of molecules. Should a near term candidate be deemed viable for development, the cost to an Investigational New Drug (IND) application is estimated to be $5 to $8 million (Collett 2005). These costs would include GMP production, preclinical toxicology by a contract house (single dose, maximally tolerated dose (MTD), dose escalation studies, animal absorption, distribution, elimination and metabolism). Standard protocols would involve preclinical toxicology under the umbrella of 7, 14, and 28 day and 3 month drug administration. The end product would be a document that would serve as an IND application.

With the successful award of an IND from the FDA, a Phase I study could be initiated in normal human volunteers and would need to include both pediatric and adult pharmacokinetic studies, including drug interactions, and evaluation in high-risk populations. These studies typically recruit 30 to 50 patients, are managed by contract research organizations and are labor intensive. A typical study would be estimated to cost $5 million. In general for any compound taken forward, detailed efficacy-defining studies leading to registration would cost $20 to $40 million each. Experts present at the workshop estimated the cost of developing a near-term compound at $75 million over 5 years. In agreement with this number, one published report estimates the average out-of-pocket clinical period costs for investigational compounds to be $60.6 million in 2000 dollars (DiMasi et al. 2003).

For long-term targets, NIAID has developed partnership grants with small biotechnology companies. The grants have averaged about $20 million, including co-support from industry, to allow a molecule to get to the IND stage.

Importantly, all of the above calculations are estimates predicated upon the rapidity at which an existing lead molecule can be advanced toward an IND. Should a previously unexplored target be chosen for drug screening, the costs assuredly will be greater. In such circumstances, the molecular biology required for drug development would significantly increase costs.

The projected cost of medication development includes only the cost for licensure and not for the subsequent manufacture and storage of the large number of treatment doses that might be required to respond to an outbreak. The development of a drug to treat poliovirus infections is not expected to be of great interest to the pharmaceutical industry. Therefore, support for this program will have to come from alternative funding sources. They could include the Bill and Melinda Gates Foundation or a new foundation dedicated specifically to the development of a polio antiviral drug as a component of the global polio eradication program. The Rotary Club does not have such a foundation in place, but it has invested over $650 million in the eradication of polio and might regard the development of an antiviral as a good backup to ensure the eventual success of its investment. Finally, consideration of support from the National Institutes of Health, the Centers for Disease Control and Prevention, and the World Health Organization is essential.

5

Implementation and Recommendations

T HE COMMITTEE RECOGNIZES THAT IDENTIFYING the resources to develop an antiviral drug against poliovirus will be challenging. Public health needs are vast and the polio eradication effort is drawing to an end with the anticipated cessation of oral poliovirus (OPV) global campaigns. The public health burden of paralytic polio that has been lifted as a result of the eradication effort has been enormous. The Global Polio Eradication Initiative estimates that over $4.6 billion has been spent on the polio eradication effort to date (Global Polio Eradication Initiative 2006). The committee thinks that it is important to ensure that past investment in the eradication effort be protected. There are two major threats to maintaining a polio-free world. First, the eradication effort involved a live vaccine that carries the risk of initiating new chains of transmission, especially in the early post-OPV years. Second, the risk of accidental or intentional release of poliovirus cannot be entirely eliminated and the consequences of such a release will grow more and more serious after routine immunization ceases.

Therefore, the committee concludes that if current plans to cease OPV administration go forward, it is important to begin development of at least one, but preferably two, polio antiviral drugs as a supplement to the tools currently available for the control of poliomyelitis outbreaks.

The successful development of antiviral drugs against poliovirus will require coordinated and sustained attention to a number of challenges: defining how the compound will be used, choosing the best targets, investing in the most promising lead compounds, determining the most appropriate approach to proving efficacy and safety and—most importantly—raising awareness of the importance of the task and mobilizing the necessary funds. Therefore, the committee recommends that a multidisciplinary steering team be assembled to guide the effort.

RECOMMENDATIONS

1. Public Health Considerations

The committee recommends that:

a. The development of one or more polio antiviral drugs should be included as a goal of the global polio eradication effort. Under the assumption that administration of OPV will eventually be halted, the availability of an effective polio antiviral will be extremely useful for outbreak control in the context of declining levels of population immunity.

b. The primary use of the antiviral/s should be to assist, possibly with IPV, in control of a cVDPV outbreak in the post-OPV era by preventing virus spread through prophylaxis of susceptible contacts and reduced virus shedding of infected persons. Treatment of patients chronically infected with poliovirus would be a secondary use of the antiviral drugs, but careful attention should be paid to the risk that resistant strains could emerge during long-term use.

c. Careful consideration should be given to plans including criteria for employment of the drug, a distribution strategy, and innovative ways of enhancing compliance.

d. Deployment of the antiviral or antiviral drugs should be under the control of public health authorities.

2. Biological Considerations

The committee recommends that:

a. Capsid-binding molecules and 3C protease inhibitors initially be given priority for consideration: the availability of promising lead compounds, the critical replication functions interrupted by these classes of compounds and the likelihood that these compounds may

thwart the emergence of resistance combine to make them the most attractive candidates for initial consideration.
b. Additional targets including $2A^{pro}$, $3D^{pol}$, 2C, 3A and RNA structures also be explored, so that information about their activity will be available if screening programs identify compounds with antipolio activity.
c. Developments in novel therapeutic approaches like siRNA, morpholinos and passive antibodies be carefully monitored; significant technological advances in these approaches could unexpectedly make one of them the most feasible and cost-effective approach to developing a polio antiviral.
d. Continued basic research into poliovirus should be encouraged. Improved understanding of the sites of replication and the development of appropriate animal models of infection, pathogenesis and shedding will make the development of a polio antiviral much more likely to succeed.

3. Developmental Considerations

The committee recommends that:

a. Compounds acting against at least two targets be developed in parallel.
b. Funding be pursued to formulate a development plan, including considering carefully the most promising compounds for development, generating realistic budget estimates, and mapping out the clinical trial and regulatory approval processes.
c. A drug development team be formed to guide the effort; the team should include public health experts (including representatives from countries where the antiviral might be tested and/or deployed), molecular biologists with expertise in poliovirus biology, clinical drug developers and industry representatives.

References

Agol, V.I. 2002. Picornavirus genome: an overview. In *Molecular Biology of Picornaviruses.* B.L. Semler and E. Wimmer, Eds. ASM Press, Washington, DC.

Alexander, J.P., Jr., H.E. Gary, Jr., and M.A. Pallansch. 1997. Duration of poliovirus excretion and its implications for acute flaccid paralysis surveillance: a review of the literature. *Journal of Infectious Diseases* 175:S176-S182.

Andino, R., G.E. Rieckhof, and D. Baltimore. 1990. A functional ribonucleoprotein complex forms around the 5' end of poliovirus RNA. *Cell* 63:369-380.

Andries, K., B. Dewindt, J. Snoeks, L. Wouters, H. Moereels, P.J. Lewi, and P.A.J. Janssen. 1990. Two groups of rhinoviruses revealed by a panel of antiviral compounds present sequence divergence and differential pathogenicity. *Journal of Virology* 64(3):1117-1123.

Andries, K., B. Dewindt, J. Snoeks, R. Willebrords, K. Van Eemeren, R. Stokbroekx, and P.A.J. Janssen. 1992. In vitro activity of pirodavir (R 77975), a substituted phenoxy-pyridazinamine with broad-spectrum antipicornaviral activity. *Antimicrobial Agents and Chemotherapy* 36(1):100-107.

Arita, M., S.L. Zhu, H. Yoshida, T. Yoneyama, T. Miyamura, and H. Shimizu. 2005. A Sabin 3-derived poliovirus recombinant contained a sequence homologous with indigenous human enterovirus species C in the viral polymerase coding region. *Journal of Virology* 79(20):12650-12657.

Arora, V., G.R. Devi, and P.L. Iversen. 2004. Neutrally charged phosphorodiamidate morpholino antisense oligomers: uptake, efficacy and pharmacokinetics. *Current Pharmaceutical Biotechnology* 5(5):431-439.

Aylward, R.B., and S.L. Cochi. 2004. Framework for evaluating the risks of paralytic poliomyelitis after global interruption of wild poliovirus transmission. *Bulletin of the World Health Organization* 82:40-46.

Aylward, R.B., R.W. Sutter, and D.L. Heymann. 2005. OPV cessation—the final step to a "polio-free" world. *Science* 310(5748):625-626.

Baltimore, D., M.F. Jacobson, J. Asso, and A.S. Huang. 1969. The formation of poliovirus proteins. *Cold Spring Harbor Symposium in Quantitative Biology* 34:741-746.

Binford, S.L., F. Maldonado, M.A. Brothers, P.T. Weady, L.S. Zalman, J.W. Meador, 3rd, D.A. Matthews, and A.K. Patick. 2005. Conservation of amino acids in human rhinovirus 3C protease correlates with broad-spectrum antiviral activity of rupintrivir, a novel human rhinovirus 3C protease inhibitor. *Antimicrobial Agents and Chemotherapy* 49(2):619-626.

Bodian, D. 1952. Experimental studies on passive immunization against poliomyelitis. II. The prophylactic effect of human gamma globulin on paralytic poliomyelitis in cynomolgus monkeys after virus feeding. *American Journal of Hygiene* 56:78-89.

Bodian, D. 1955. Emerging concept of poliomyelitis infection. *Science* 122:105.

Bodian, D., and D.M. Horstmann. 1965. Polioviruses. In *Viral and Rickettsial Infections of Man,* fourth ed. F.L. Horsfall, Jr. and I. Tamm, Eds. J.B. Lippincott, Philadelphia.

Carr, J., J. Ives, L. Kelly, R. Lambkin, J. Oxford, D. Mendel, L. Tai, and N. Roberts. 2002. Influenza virus carrying neuraminidase with reduced sensitivity to oseltamivir carboxylate has altered properties in vitro and is compromised for infectivity and replicative ability in vivo. *Antiviral Research* 54(2):79-88.

CDC (Centers for Disease Control and Prevention). 2005a. Conclusions and recommendations of the advisory committee on poliomyelitis eradication—Geneva, Switzerland, October 2005. *Morbidity and Mortality Weekly Report* 54(46):1186-1188.

CDC. 2005b. Poliovirus infections in four unvaccinated children—Minnesota, August-October 2005. *Morbidity and Mortality Weekly Report* 54(41):1053-1055.

Census Bureau, Population Division, International Programs Center. 2005. IDB Summary Demographic Data. Accessed online 12/16/05 at http://www.census.gov/ipc/www/idbsum.html.

Coffin, J.M. 1995. HIV population dynamics in vivo: implications for genetic variation, pathogenesis, and therapy. *Science* 267(5197):483-489.

Collett, M.S. 2005. Capsid inhibitors: a path to polio antiviral drugs. Presented at the Workshop on Development of a Polio Antiviral, National Research Council, November 1, 2005, Washington, DC.

Crotty, S., D. Maag, J.J. Arnold, W. Zhong, J.Y. Lau, Z. Hong, R. Andino, and C.E. Cameron. 2000. The broad-spectrum antiviral ribonucleoside ribavirin is an RNA virus mutagen. *Nature Medicine* 6(12):1375-1379. Erratum in: *Nature Medicine* 7(2):255.

Crowder, S., and K. Kirkegaard. 2005. Trans-dominant inhibition of RNA viral replication can slow growth of drug-resistant viruses. *Nature Genetics* 37(7):665-666.

de la Torre, J.C., E. Wimmer, and J.J. Holland. 1990. Very high frequency of reversion to guanidine resistance in clonal pools of guanidine-dependent type 1 poliovirus. *Journal of Virology* 64(2):664-667.

DiMasi, J.A., R.W. Hansen, and H.G. Grabowski. 2003. The price of innovation: new estimates of drug development costs. *Journal of Health Economics* 22:151-185.

Domingo, E., J. Holland, and P. Ahlquist. 1988. *RNA Genetics.* CRC Press, Boca Raton.

Duintjer Tebbens, R.J., M.A. Pallansch, O.M. Kew, V.M. Caceres, R.W. Sutter, and K.M. Thompson. 2005. A dynamic model of poliomyelitis outbreaks: learning from the past to help inform the future. *American Journal of Epidemiology* 162(4):358-372.

Egger, D., R. Gosert, and K. Bienz. 2002. Role of cellular structures in viral RNA replication. In *Molecular Biology of Picornaviruses*. B.L. Semler and E. Wimmer, Eds. ASM Press, Washington, DC.

Eigen, M. 1993. Viral quasispecies. *Scientific American* 269(1):42-49.

Fairbrother, R.W., and E.W. Hurst. 1930. The pathogenesis of experimental poliomyelitis. *Journal of Pathology and Bacteriology* 33:17-45.

Fenner, F., D.A. Henderon, I. Arita, Z. Jezek, and I.D. Ladnyi. 1988. Smallpox and its eradication. World Health Organization, Geneva.

Filman, D.J., R. Syed, M. Chow, A.J. Macadam, P.D. Minor, and J.M. Hogle. 1989. Structural factors that control conformational transitions and serotype specificity in type 3 poliovirus. *The EMBO Journal* 8:1567-1579.

Flanegan, J.B., and D. Baltimore. 1977. Poliovirus-specific primer-dependent RNA polymerase able to copy poly(A). *Proceedings of the National Academy of Sciences of the United States of America* 74(9):3677-3680.

Franco, D., H.B. Pathak, C.E. Cameron, B. Rombaut, E. Wimmer, and A.V. Paul. 2005. Stimulation of poliovirus RNA synthesis and virus maturation in a HeLa cell-free in vitro translation-RNA replication system by viral protein 3CD^pro. *Virology Journal* 2:86.

Frank, R.G. 2003. New estimates of drug development costs. *Journal of Health Economics* 22:325-330.

Gitlin, L., S. Karelsky, and R. Andino. 2002. Short interfering RNA confers intracellular antiviral immunity in human cells. *Nature* 418:430-434.

Global Polio Eradication Initiative. 2006. Donor Contributions and Projections to Polio Eradication 1985-2008. Accessed online 2/16/06 at http://www.polioeradication.org/content/general/HistContributionWebJan06.pdf.

Gnann, J.W., Jr., C.S. Crumpacker, J.P. Lalezari, J.A. Smith, S.K. Tyring, K.F. Baum, M.J. Borucki, W.P. Joseph, G.J. Mertz, R.T. Steigbigel, G.A. Cloud, S.J. Soong, L.C. Sherrill, D.A. DeHertogh, and R.J. Whitley. 1998. Sorivudine versus acyclovir for treatment of dermatomal herpes zoster in human immunodeficiency virus-infected patients: results from a randomized, controlled clinical trial. *Antimicrobial Agents and Chemotherapy* 42(5):1139-1145.

Grant, R.A., C.N. Hiremath, D.J. Filman, R. Syed, K. Andries, and J.M. Hogle. 1994. Structures of poliovirus complexes with anti viral drugs: implications for viral stability and drug design. *Current Biology* 4(9):784-797.

Halsey, N.A., J. Pinto, F. Espinosa-Rosales, M.A. Faure-Fontenla, E. da Silva, A.J. Khan, A.D.B. Webster, P. Minor, G. Dunn, E. Asturias, H. Hussain, M.A. Pallansch, O.M. Kew, J. Winkelstein, R. Sutter, and the Polio Project Team. 2004. Search for poliovirus carriers among people with primary immune deficiency diseases in the United States, Mexico, Brazil and the United Kingdom. *Bulletin of the World Health Organization* 82:3-8.

Hellen, C.U., M. Facke, H.G. Krausslich, C.K. Lee, and E. Wimmer. 1991. Characterization of poliovirus 2A proteinase by mutational analysis: residues required for autocatalytic activity are essential for induction of cleavage of eukaryotic initiation factor 4F polypeptide p220. *Journal of Virology* 65(8):4226-4231.

Hiremath, C.N., R.A. Grant, D.J. Filman, and J.M. Hogle. 1995. Binding of the antiviral drug WIN51711 to the Sabin strain of type 3 poliovirus: structural comparison with drug binding in rhinovirus 14. *Acta Crystallographica Section D-Biological Crystallography* 51(4):473-489.

Hiremath, C.N., D.J. Filman, R.A. Grant, and J.M. Hogle. 1997. Ligand-induced conformational changes in poliovirus-antiviral drug complexes. *Acta Crystallographica Section D-Biological Crystallography* 53(5):558-570.

Hirst, G. 1962. Genetic recombination with Newcastle disease virus, polioviruses, and influenza. Cold Spring Harbor Symposium. *Quantitative Biology* 27:303-308.

Hogle, J.M., M. Chow, and D.J. Filman. 1985. Three-dimensional structure of poliovirus at 2.9 A resolution. *Science* 229:1358-1365.

Holland, J., K. Spindler, F. Horodyski, E. Grabau, S. Nichol, and S. VandePol. 1982. Rapid evolution of RNA genomes. *Science* 215(4540):1577-1585.

Holland, J.J., J.C. de la Torre, and D.A. Steinhauer. 1992. RNA virus populations as quasispecies. *Current Topics in Microbiology and Immunology* 176:1-20.

Horie, H., S. Koike, T. Kurata, Y. Sato-Yoshida, I. Ise, Y. Ota, S. Abe, K. Hioki, H. Kato, and C. Taya. 1994. Transgenic mice carrying the human poliovirus receptor: new animal models for study of poliovirus neurovirulence. *Journal of Virology* 68:681-688.

Horstmann, D.M., R. Ward, and J.L. Melnick. 1946. The isolation of poliomyelitis virus from human extra-neural sources. III. Persistence of virus in stools after acute infection. *Journal of Clinical Investigation* 25:278-283.

Jackson, W.T., T.H. Giddings, Jr., M.P. Taylor, S. Mulinyawe, M. Rabinovitch, R.R. Kopito, and K. Kirkegaard. 2005. Subversion of cellular autophagosomal machinery by RNA viruses. *PLoS Biology* 3(5):e156.

Joseph-McCarthy, D., S.K. Tsang, D.J. Filman, J.M. Hogle, and M. Karplus. 2001. Use of MCSS to design small targeted libraries: application to picornavirus ligands. *Journal of the American Chemical Society* 123(51):12758-12769.

Kew, O.M., R.W. Sutter, B.K. Nottay, M.J. McDonough, D.R. Prevots, L. Quick, and M.A. Pallansch. 1998. Prolonged replication of a type 1 vaccine-derived poliovirus in an immunodeficient patient. *Journal of Clinical Microbiology* 36:2893-2899.

Kew, O., V. Morris-Glasgow, M. Landaverde, C. Burns, J. Shaw, Z. Garib, J. Andre, E. Blackman, C.J. Freeman, J. Jorba, R. Sutter, G. Tambini, L. Venczel, C. Pedreira, F. Laender, H. Shimizu, T. Yoneyama, T. Miyamura, H. van Der Avoort, M.S. Oberste, D. Kilpatrick, S. Cochi, M. Pallansch, and C. de Quadros. 2002. Outbreak of poliomyelitis in Hispaniola associated with circulating type 1 vaccine-derived poliovirus. *Science* 296:356-359.

Kew, O.M., P.F. Wright, V.I. Agol, F. Delpeyroux, H. Shimizu, N. Nathanson, and M.A. Pallansch. 2004. Circulating vaccine-derived polioviruses: current state of knowledge. *Bulletin of the World Health Organization* 82(1):16-23.

Kew, O.M., R.W. Sutter, E.M. de Gourville, W.R. Dowdle, and M.A. Pallansch. 2005. Vaccine-derived polioviruses and the endgame strategy for global polio eradication. *Annual Review of Microbiology* 59:587-635.

Kirkegaard, K., and D. Baltimore. 1986. The mechanism of RNA recombination in poliovirus. *Cell* 47:433-443.

Kitamura, N., B.L. Semler, P.G. Rothberg, G.R. Larsen, C.J. Adler, A.J. Dorner, E.A. Emini, R. Hanecak, J.J. Lee, S. van der Werf, C.W. Anderson, and E. Wimmer. 1981. Primary structure, gene organization and polypeptide expression of poliovirus RNA. *Nature* 291(5816):547-553.

Koike, S., H. Horie, I. Ise, A. Okitsu, M. Yoshida, N. Iizuka, K. Takeuchi, T. Takegami, and A. Nomoto. 1990. The poliovirus receptor protein is produced both as membrane-bound and secreted forms. *EMBO Journal* 9:3217-3224.

Kuechler, E., J. Seipelt, H.D. Liebig, and W. Sommergruber. 2002. Picornavirus-mediated proteinase shut-off of host cell translation: direct cleavage of a cellular initiation factor. In *Molecular Biology of Picornaviruses*. B.L. Semler and E. Wimmer, Eds. ASM Press, Washington, DC.

Lentz, K.N., A.D. Smith, S.C. Geisler, S. Cox, P. Buontempo, A. Skelton, J. Demartino, E. Rozhon, J. Schwartz, V. Girijavallabhan, J. O'Connell, and E. Arnold. 1997. Structure of poliovirus type 2 Lansing complexed with antiviral agent SCH48973: comparison of the structural and biological properties of three poliovirus serotypes. *Structure* 5(7):961-978.

Leong, L.E.C., C.T. Cornell, and B.L. Semler. 2002. Processing determinants and functions of cleavage products of picornavirus proteins. In *Molecular Biology of Picornaviruses*. B.L. Semler and E. Wimmer, Eds. ASM Press, Washington, DC.

MacLennan, C., G. Dunn, A.P. Huissoon, D.S. Kumararatne, J. Martin, P. O'Leary, R.A. Thompson, H. Osman, P. Wood, P. Minor, D.J. Wood, and D. Pillay. 2004. Failure to clear persistent vaccine-derived neurovirulent poliovirus infection in an immuno-deficient man. *Lancet* 363:1509-1513.

Martin, J., K. Odoom, G. Tuite, G. Dunn, N. Hopewell, G. Cooper, C. Fitzharris, K. Butler, W.W. Hall, and P.D. Minor. 2004. Long-term excretion of vaccine-derived poliovirus by a healthy child. *Journal of Virology* 78:13839-13847.

Melnick, J.L. 1996. Enteroviruses: polioviruses, coxsackieviruses, echoviruses, and newer enteroviruses, vol. 1. In *Virology*, third ed. B.N. Fields, Ed. Raven Press, New York.

Mendelsohn, C.L., E. Wimmer, and V.R. Racaniello. 1989. Cellular receptor for poliovirus: molecular cloning, nucleotide sequence, and expression of a new member of the immunoglobulin super family. *Cell* 56:855-865.

Minor, P. 1997. Poliovirus. In *Viral Pathogenesis*. N. Nathanson, Ed. Lippincott-Raven, Philadelphia.

Molla A., A.V. Paul, and E. Wimmer. 1991. Cell-free, de novo synthesis of poliovirus. *Science* 254(5038):1647-1651.

Molla, A., A.V. Paul, M. Schmid, S.K. Jang, and E. Wimmer. 1993. Studies on dicistronic polioviruses implicate viral proteinase 2A^{pro} in RNA replication. *Virology* 196(2):739-747.

Mosimann, S.C., M.M. Cherney, S. Sia, S. Plotch, and M.N. James. 1997. Refined X-ray crystallographic structure of the poliovirus 3C gene product. *Journal of Molecular Biology* 273(5):1032-1047.

Mueller, S., E. Wimmer, and J. Cello. 2005. Poliovirus and poliomyelitis: a tale of guts, brains, and an accidental event. *Virus Research* 111:175-193.

Nathanson, N. 2005. David Bodian's contribution to the development of poliovirus vaccine. *American Journal of Epidemiology* 161:207-212.

Nathanson, N., and J.R. Martin. 1979. The epidemiology of poliomyelitis: enigmas surrounding its appearance, epidemicity, and disappearance. *American Journal of Epidemiology* 110(6):672-692.

Nicklin, M.J., K.S. Harris, P.V. Pallai, and E. Wimmer. 1988. Poliovirus proteinase 3C: large-scale expression, purification, and specific cleavage activity on natural and synthetic substrates in vitro. *Journal of Virology* 62(12):4586-4593.

Olsen, D.B., A.B. Eldrup, L. Bartholomew, B. Bhat, M.R. Bosserman, A. Ceccacci, L.F. Colwell, J.F. Fay, O.A. Flores, K.L. Getty, J.A. Grobler, R.L. LaFemina, E.J. Markel, G. Migliaccio, M. Prhavc, M.W. Stahlhut, J.E. Tomassini, M. MacCoss, D.J. Hazuda, and S.S. Carroll. 2004. A 7-deaza-adenosine analog is a potent and selective inhibitor of hepatitis C virus replication with excellent pharmacokinetic properties. *Antimicrobial Agents and Chemotherapy* 48(10):3944-3953.

Parsley, T.B., J.S. Towner, L.B. Blyn, E. Ehrenfeld, and B.L. Semler. 1997. Poly (rC) binding protein 2 forms a ternary complex with the 5'-terminal sequences of poliovirus RNA and the viral 3CD proteinase. *RNA* 3(10):1124-1134.

Patick, A.K., S.L. Binford, M.A. Brothers, R.L. Jackson, C.E. Ford, M.D. Diem, F. Maldonado, P.S. Dragovich, R. Zhou, T.J. Prins, S.A. Fuhrman, J.W. Meador, L.S. Zalman, D.A. Matthews, and S.T. Worland. 1999. In vitro antiviral activity of AG7088, a potent inhibitor of human rhinovirus 3C protease. *Antimicrobial Agents and Chemotherapy* 43:2444-2450.

Patick, A.K., M.A. Brothers, F. Maldonado, S. Binford, O. Maldonado, S. Fuhrman, A. Petersen, G.J. Smith 3rd, L.S. Zalman, L.A. Burns-Naas, and J.Q. Tran. 2005. In vitro antiviral activity and single-dose pharmacokinetics in humans of a novel, orally bioavailable inhibitor of human rhinovirus 3C protease. *Antimicrobial Agents and Chemotherapy* 49:2267-2275.

Paul, A. 2002. Possible unifying mechanism of picornavirus genome replication. In *Molecular Biology of Picornaviruses*. B.L. Semler and E. Wimmer, Eds. ASN Press, Washington, DC.

Paul, A.V., J.H. van Boom, D. Filippov, and E. Wimmer. 1998. Protein primed RNA synthesis by purified poliovirus RNA polymerase. *Nature* 393(6682):280-284.

Paul, A.V., E. Rieder, D.W. Kim, J.H. van Boom, and E. Wimmer. 2000. Identification of an RNA hairpin in poliovirus RNA that serves as the primary template in the in vitro uridylylation of VPg. *Journal of Virology* 74(22):10359-10370.

Petersen, J.F., M.M. Cherney, H.D. Liebig, T. Skern, E. Kuechler, and M.N. James. 1999. The structure of the 2A proteinase from a common cold virus: a proteinase responsible for the shut-off of host-cell protein synthesis. *EMBO Journal* 18(20):5463-5475.

Pfeiffer, J.K., and K. Kirkegaard. 2005. Increased fidelity reduces poliovirus fitness and virulence under selective pressure in mice. *PLoS Pathogens* 1(2):e11.

Pfister, T., and E. Wimmer. 1999. Characterization of the nucleoside triphosphatase activity of poliovirus protein 2C reveals a mechanism by which guanidine inhibits poliovirus replication. *Journal of Biological Chemistry* 274(11):6992-7001.

Racaniello, V. 2001. Picornaviridae: the viruses and their replication. In *Field Virology*. P. Howley and D. Knipe, Eds. Lippinkott, Williams and Wilkins, Philadelphia.

Racaniello, V.R., and D. Baltimore. 1981. Molecular cloning of poliovirus cDNA and determination of the complete nucleotide sequence of the viral genome. *Proceedings of the National Academy of Sciences of the United States of America* 78:4887.

Reichert, J.M. 2001. Monoclonal antibodies and the clinic. *Nature Biotechnology* 19:819-822.

Rinaldo, C.R. 2005. Passive immunization against poliomyelitis: the Hammon gamma globulin field trials, 1951-1953. *American Journal of Public Health* 95(5):790-799.

Romanova, L.I., E.A. Talskaya, M.S. Kolesnikova, and V.I. Agol. 1980. Biochemical evidence for intertypic genetic recombination of poliovirus. *FEBS Letters* 118:109-112.

Rossmann, M.G. 2002. Picornavirus structure overview. In *Molecular Biology of Picornaviruses*. B.L. Semler and E. Wimmer, Eds. ASM Press, Washington, DC.

Rossmann, M.G., J. Bella, P.R. Kolatkar, Y. He, E. Wimmer, R.J. Kuhn, and T.S. Baker. 2000. Cell recognition and entry by rhino- and enteroviruses. *Virology* 269:239-247.

Sabin, A.B. 1956. Pathogenesis of poliomyelitis; reappraisal in the light of new data. *Science* 123:1151-1157.

Sabin, A., and R. Ward. 1941. Nature of non-paralytic and transitory paralytic poliomyelitis in rhesus monkeys inoculated with human virus. *Journal of Experimental Medicine* 73:757-770.

Semler, B.L., and E. Wimmer, Eds. 2002. *Molecular Biology of Picornaviruses*. ASM Press, Washington, DC.

Simoes, E.A.F, B. Padmini, M.C. Steinhoff, M. Jadhav, and T.J. John. 1985. Antibody response of infants to two doses of inactivated poliovirus vaccine of enhanced potency. *American Journal of Diseases of Children* 139:977-980.

Skern, T., B. Hampölz, A. Guarne, I. Fita, E. Bergmann, J. Petersen, and M.N.G. James. 2002. Structure and function of picornavirus proteinases. In *Molecular Biology of Picornaviruses*. B.L. Semler and E. Wimmer, Eds. ASM Press, Washington, DC.

Sormunen, H., M. Stenvik, J. Eskola, and T. Hovi. 2004. Age- and dose-interval-dependent antibody responses to inactivated poliovirus vaccine. *Journal of Medical Virology* 63:305-310.

Stanway, G., T. Hovi, N.G. Knowles. 2002. Hyppiä. Molecular and biological basis of picornavirus taxonomy. In *Molecular Biology of Picornaviruses*. B.L. Semler and E. Wimmer, Eds. ASM Press, Washington, DC.

Sutter, R. 2005. Antiviral compounds for polio eradication. Presented at the Workshop on Development of a Polio Antiviral, National Research Council, November 1, 2005, Washington, DC.

Svitkin, Y.V., A.E. Gorbalenya, Y.A. Kazachkov, and V.I. Agol. 1979. Encephalomyocarditis virus-specific polypepride p22 possessing a proteolytic activity: preliminary mapping on the viral genome. *FEBS Letters* 108:6-9.

Thompson, A.A., and O.B. Peersen. 2004. Structural basis for proteolysis-dependent activation of the poliovirus RNA-dependent RNA polymerase. *EMBO Journal* 23(17):3462-3471.

Tolskaya, E., L. Romanova, W. Kolesnikova, and V.I. Agol. 1983. Intertypic recombination in poliovirus: genetic and biochemical studies. *Virology* 123:121-132.

Toyoda, H., M.J. Nicklin, M.G. Murray, C.W. Anderson, J.J. Dunn, F.W. Studier, and E. Wimmer. 1986. A second virus-encoded proteinase involved in proteolytic processing of poliovirus polyprotein. *Cell* 45:761-770.

Vignuzzi, M., J.K. Stone, and R. Andino. 2005. Ribavirin and lethal mutagenesis of poliovirus: molecular mechanisms, resistance and biological implications. *Virus Research* 107(2):173-181.

Weidman, M.K., R. Sharma, S. Raychaudhuri, P. Kundu, W. Tsai, and A. Dasgupta. 2003. The interaction of cytoplasmic RNA viruses with the nucleus. *Virus Research* 95(1-2):75-85.

Wenner, H.A., A. Kamitsuka, M. Lenahan, and I. Archetti. 1959. The pathogenesis of polio-myelitis, site of multiplication of poliovirus in cynomolgus monkeys after alimentary infection. *Archiv fur die Gesamte Virusforschung* 9:537-558.

WHO (World Health Organization). Polio Weekly Global Update, December 21, 2005. WHO, Geneva.

Wimmer, E., C.U.T. Hellen, and X. Cao. 1993. Genetics of poliovirus. *Annual Review of Genetics* 273:353-436.

Wu, J.Z., N. Yao, M. Walker, and Z. Hong. 2005. Recent advances in discovery and development of promising therapeutics against hepatitis C virus NS5B RNA-dependent RNA polymerase. *Mini Reviews in Medicinal Chemistry* 5(12):1103-1112.

Yang, Y., R. Rijnbrand, S. Watowich, and S.M. Lemon. 2004. Genetic evidence for an interaction between a picornaviral cis-acting RNA replication element and 3CD protein. *Journal of Biological Chemistry* 279(13):12659-12667.

Yeung, M.L., Y. Bennasser, S.Y. Le, and K.T. Jeang. 2005. siRNA, miRNA and HIV: promises and challenges. *Cell Research* 15(11-12):935-946.

Ypma-Wong, M.F., P.G. Dewalt, V.H. Johnson, J.G. Lamb, and B.L. Semler. 1988. Protein 3CD is the major poliovirus proteinase responsible for cleavage of the P1 capsid precursor. *Virology* 166:265-270.

Appendixes

Appendix A

Statement of Task

An ad hoc committee will produce a consensus report on the development of polio antivirals as a potential element of the Global Polio Eradication Initiative. The report will address the following issues:

- The feasibility and appropriateness of using a polio antiviral drug in the post-eradication era
- The properties a polio antiviral compound would need in order to meet the goals of the eradication program
- The most promising targets for polio antiviral drug development
- A comparison of different approaches to polio antiviral drug development, including an assessment of the required scientific expertise, infrastructural needs, risks, obstacles, and relative costs

As appropriate, the committee will make recommendations on whether and how to proceed with the development of a polio antiviral.

Appendix B

Committee Biographical Sketches

Samuel L. Katz, Chair, is the Wilburt Cornell Davison Professor and Chairman emeritus of Pediatrics at Duke University. Following his medical training at Harvard University, pediatrics residency, and a research fellowship in virology and infectious diseases, he became a staff member at Children's Hospital working with Nobel laureate John F. Enders. During his 12 years with Enders, they developed the attenuated measles virus vaccine now used worldwide. Katz' career has been devoted to infectious disease research focusing principally on vaccine research, development and policy. In addition to his investigations of measles, he has been involved in studies of vaccinia, polio, rubella, influenza, pertussis, haemophilus influenzae b conjugates, HIV and others. Dr. Katz has received many honors including the Howland Medal of the American Pediatric Society and the Gold Medal of the Sabin Vaccine Institute, and was elected to the Institute of Medicine in 1982. He currently chairs the Board of the International Vaccine Institute in Seoul, Korea, and, in the past, chaired the Committee on Infectious Diseases of the American Academy of Pediatrics (Redbook Committee), the Advisory Committee on Immunization Practices (ACIP) of the CDC, the Vaccine Priorities Study of the Institute of Medicine (IOM), and several WHO, CVI and NIH panels. He has also chaired the Public Policy Council of the Infectious Diseases Society of America (IDSA) and currently co-chairs its National Network for Immunization Information.

Raul Andino is Professor of Microbiology and Immunology at the University of California, San Francisco (UCSF). Dr. Andino joined the Department of Microbiology and Immunology at the University of California, San Francisco in 1992 and began a program to develop RNA viruses as vaccine vectors. His laboratory is interested in the fundamental questions of how viruses cause disease and how the host defends itself against viruses. He has continued an intensive investigation of RNA virus replication and has discovered an important connection between viral replication and viral translation. More recently, his laboratory has begun investigating the potential use of RNA mutagens and RNA interference as antiviral drugs. Dr. Andino has published over 50 papers in prestigious journals, co-directs a graduate course in animal viruses at UCSF, is a member of the editorial boards of the *Journal of Virology* and *Virology*, and is the recipient of an Eli Lilly award in microbiological research and a Science Award from the Cancer Federation. Dr. Andino has served on numerous advisory committees to the NIH including study sections and strategic planning for the AIDS vaccine program at NIAID. He received his B.S. in Microbiology and his Ph.D. in Chemistry from the University of Buenos Aires. He completed his postdoctoral work with Nobel laureate David Baltimore at the Whitehead Institute, MIT and at Rockefeller University from 1986-1992.

Diane Joseph-McCarthy is a Principal Research Scientist in the Structural Biology and Computational Chemistry Division of the Chemical and Screening Sciences Department at Wyeth Research. Her research interests are in the general area of molecular recognition and include virtual screening, structure-based drug design, and computational methods. Dr. Joseph-McCarthy received her bachelor degree in Chemistry with a minor in Computer Science from Boston University and her doctorate degree in Physical Chemistry from MIT. While at MIT, she worked with Professors Gregory A. Petsko and Martin Karplus (Harvard University) and used computational approaches to study the reactivity of the enzyme triosephosphate isomerase. Following her Ph.D. dissertation, she was a Research Fellow in the Department of Biological Chemistry and Molecular Pharmacology at Harvard Medical School. This research involved the use and development of new computational methods for the design of small combinatorial libraries of capsid-binding ligands for poliovirus and the related rhinovirus. Dr. Joseph-McCarthy has been the recipient of postdoctoral fellowships from the Radcliffe Bunting Institute, the Charles A. King Medical Foundation, and the Giovanni Armenise-Harvard Foundation. She has more than 30 publications, several patents, and has given numerous invited talks.

John F. Modlin is Professor of Pediatrics and Medicine, Chairman of the Department of Pediatrics at Dartmouth Medical School, and Medical Director of the Children's Hospital at Dartmouth. He is also a member of the Infectious Disease Section at the Dartmouth-Hitchcock Medical Center in Lebanon, New Hampshire. He received both his A.B. and M.D. degrees from Duke University. His pediatric internship and residency were performed at the Children's Hospital in Boston between 1971 and 1973, including a year at St. Mary's Hospital in London. After 2 years of service with the Epidemic Intelligence Service at the Centers for Disease Control and Prevention, he returned to Boston in 1975 to complete his residency and infectious disease fellowship. From 1978 to 1983 he was Instructor and Assistant Professor of Pediatrics at Harvard Medical School and physician at the Children's Hospital in Boston. He moved to Johns Hopkins in 1983 where he headed the Pediatric AIDS Program and continued his research on enterovirus diseases. He has been at Dartmouth since 1991. Dr. Modlin's research interests include perinatal viral infections, pathophysiology of enterovirus infections, and poliovirus immunization. He has authored or co-authored more than 200 papers in the medical literature on these or related topics. Dr. Modlin has served as Vice-Chair of the Pediatric AIDS Clinical Trials Group Executive Committee and as a Chair of the FDA Antiviral Drugs Advisory Committee, and Chair of the CDC Advisory Committee on Immunization Practices.

Neal Nathanson is Associate Dean for Global Health Programs at the University of Pennsylvania Medical Center. In July 2003, Dr. Nathanson retired as Vice Provost for Research at the University of Pennsylvania, responsible for oversight of the whole research enterprise of the University, having served since December 2000. From July 1998 to September 2000, Dr. Nathanson served as Director of the Office of AIDS Research (OAR) at the National Institutes of Health responsible for coordinating the scientific, budgetary, legislative, and policy components of the NIH AIDS research programs, as well as for promoting collaborative research activities in domestic and international settings. Dr. Nathanson was educated at Harvard University, where he received both a B.S. and an M.D., followed by clinical training in internal medicine at the University of Chicago and postdoctoral training in virology at the Johns Hopkins University. Early in his career, Dr. Nathanson spent 2 years at the Centers for Disease Control and Prevention, where he headed the Poliomyelitis Surveillance Unit. Later, he joined the faculty of the Johns Hopkins Schools of Medicine and Public Health, where he became Professor and head of the Division of Infectious Diseases in the Department of Epidemiology. He then moved to the University of Pennsylvania where he chaired the Department of Microbiology for 15 years, finally serving for 2 years as Vice Dean for Research and Research Training. Dr. Nathanson is particularly known for his contributions to the field of viral pathogenesis, having edited the definitive text on this subject. He has also made significant contributions to the epidemiology of viral diseases.

Richard J. Whitley is Professor of Pediatrics at the University of Alabama at Birmingham. He completed his undergraduate studies at Duke University. He completed medical school at George Washington University and completed a postdoctoral fellowship at the University of Alabama at Birmingham. During postdoctoral training he developed an interest in pursuing molecular pathogenesis of herpes simplex virus infections. These studies have been extended to collaboration with investigators at the University of Chicago through joint program projects. In addition, he is responsible for the National Institute of Allergy and Infectious Diseases Collaborative Antiviral Study Group, a multicenter collaboration of investigators attempting to improve the treatment of human herpes simplex and varicella zoster infections.

Eckard Wimmer is a Distinguished Professor at Stony Brook University School of Medicine. Born in Berlin, Germany, in 1936, Wimmer received the *doctor rerum naturalium* in Organic Chemistry in Goettingen, Germany, in 1962. Being intrigued by the chemistry of living cells, he switched his research interests first to biochemistry at the University of British Columbia, Vancouver, in 1964, then to virology at the University of Illinois, Urbana, in 1966. Wimmer started his academic career as an Assistant Professor of Microbiology at St. Louis University, St. Louis, in 1968, where he began to study poliovirus, a system that became the scientific challenge of his life. In 1974, he joined the Department of Microbiology at Stony Brook University where he served as Chairperson from 1984 to 1999. In 2002 he was promoted to the rank of Distinguished Professor. Dr. Wimmer has always looked at viruses as biological entities that replicate and can cause disease, on the one hand, and as aggregates of organic compounds, on the other. His research therefore focuses on mechanisms of pathogenesis and the (bio)chemistry of poliovirus. The latter has led his research group to succeed in the cell-free chemical/biochemical synthesis of poliovirus in the absence of natural template. Dr. Wimmer has authored over 300 publications of which several described landmarks in virology.

Appendix C

Workshop Agenda and Participant List

November 1-2, 2005
Keck Center of the National Academies
500 Fifth Street, N.W. • Washington, D.C.

AGENDA

Tuesday, November 1, 2005

8:00 a.m.   Continental Breakfast

8:30 a.m.   **Committee orientation (closed session)**

9:00 a.m.   **Workshop convocation and introductions –**
            Samuel Katz, chairman

9:30 a.m.   **Polio eradication plan update**
            Looking ahead to the end-game: *Bruce Aylward*
            Strategies for the OPV cessation era: *Roland Sutter*
            Potential roles for an antiviral: *Mark Pallansch*

10:15 a.m. **Overview of poliovirus biology and pathogenesis**
            Eckard Wimmer

10:45 a.m. Coffee Break

11:00 a.m. **Introduction to potential targets**
Mutagenesis and RNAi: *Raul Andino*
Capsid-binding compounds: *Marc Collett*
Exploiting dominant inhibition: *Karla Kirkegaard*
Protease inhibitors: *Amy Patick*

12:00 p.m. **Organization of afternoon breakout sessions**

12:30 p.m. Buffet Lunch

1:30 p.m. **Breakout sessions**

3:30 p.m. Coffee Break

3:45 p.m. **Reports on breakout sessions and discussion**

5:30 p.m. Adjourn

Wednesday, November 2, 2005

8:00 a.m. Continental Breakfast

8:30 a.m. **Organization of day 2 breakout groups**

9:00 a.m. **Working breakout group discussions**
1. Public Health group: How would the drug be used in eradication? Who would patients be, how would they be identified and reached? What would be the advantages and disadvantages of the potential compounds identified in day 1 for different aspects of eradication?
2. Biology group: Evaluate each of the potential antivirals: how difficult would each be to develop, how likely to elicit resistance, how long would it take to develop, what would be its possible safety issues?
3. Development group: How much would each type of antiviral cost to develop? How hard might it be to move them

> **through the approval process? Who might develop them?
> What are the likely timelines involved for each? What are
> possible sources of funding?**

10:30 a.m. Coffee Break

10:45 a.m. **Report from breakout group 1 and discussion**

11:30 p.m. **Report from breakout group 2 and discussion**

12:15 p.m. Lunch

1:15 p.m. **Report from breakout group 3 and discussion**

2:00 p.m. **Wrap-up: Designing and filling in a decision matrix for
each compound**

4:00 p.m. Adjourn

PARTICIPANT LIST

Jim Alexander, *CDC*
Bruce Aylward, *WHO*
Debra Birnkrant, *Center for Drug Evaluation and Research, FDA*
Craig Cameron, *Pennsylvania State University*
Marc Collett, *ViroDefense, Inc.*
Walter Dowdle, *The Task Force for Child Survival and Development*
Ellie Ehrenfeld, *NIAID, NIH*
Diane Griffin, *Johns Hopkins Bloomberg School of Public Health*
Matthias Gromeier, *Duke University Medical Center*
Neal Halsey, *Johns Hopkins Bloomberg School of Public Health*
Stephen Hughes, *National Cancer Institute*
Kristin Kenyan, *CDC*
Karla Kirkegaard, *Stanford University School of Medicine*
Mauricio Landaverde, *Pan American Health Organization*
Catherine Laughlin, *NIAID, NIH*
Mark McKinlay, *Gentara Corporation*
Philip Minor, *National Institute for Biological Standards and Control, UK*

Akhter Molla, *Abbott Laboratories*
Mark Pallansch, *CDC*
Amy Patick, *Pfizer*
Olve Peersen, *Colorado State University*
Jane Seward, *CDC*
Tim Skern, *Medical University of Vienna*
Roland Sutter, *WHO*
Kimberly Thompson, *Harvard School of Public Health*
Linda Venczel, *CDC*
Margie Watkins, *CDC*
Jerry Winkelstein, *Johns Hopkins Children's Center*
Peter Wright, *Vanderbilt University School of Medicine*

Staff from the National Academies Board on Life Sciences

Ann Reid, *Study Director*
Anne Jurkowski, *Program Assistant*
Fran Sharples, *Director, Board on Life Sciences*